GW01091221

CANNABIS OIL

CURED

MY

CANCER

John Gabriel (Mc Donald)

Copyright 2017

ISBN: 978-0-9958881-1-1

Dedicated to victims of cancer and those committed to discovering and promoting the healing of cancer through the wonders of nature.

Special thanks to my good friends Criss and Jessa of Farm Assist Medical Cannabis Dispensary, Halifax, Nova Scotia, Canada for their support and contribution of cannabis oil that undoubtedly cured my canccr. It was these good people who stood with me and steered me in the direction of good food and towards the healing world of cannabis oil and Essiac Tea, both of which were instrumental in the healing of my cancer. Indeed, I owe them my life. Other well meaning friends told me in no uncertain terms to follow the doctor's advice. I quietly declined. Thank God I did.

GENERAL QUOTES ON MEDICAL USE

OF CANNABIS AND PROHIBITION

HON. FRANCIS YOUNG DEA ADMINISTRATIVE LAW JUDGE – 1988:

*"In strict medical terms marijuana is far safer than many foods we commonly consume. For example, eating 10 raw potatoes can result in a toxic response. By comparison, it is physically impossible to eat enough marijuana to induce death. Marijuana in its natural form is **one of the safest therapeutically active substances known to man**. By any measure of rational analysis marijuana can be safely used within the supervised routine of medical care."*

Sep. 6, 1988 ruling in the matter of "Marijuana Rescheduling Petition"

DR. JOYCELYN ELDERS, MD, FORMER US SURGEON GENERAL:

*"The evidence is overwhelming that marijuana can relieve certain types of pain, nausea, vomiting and other symptoms caused by such illnesses as multiple sclerosis, cancer and AIDS — or by the harsh drugs sometimes used to treat them. And it can do so with remarkable safety. Indeed, **marijuana is less toxic than many of the drugs that physicians prescribe every day.**"*

DR. SANJAY GUPTA:

"I mistakenly believed the Drug Enforcement Agency listed marijuana as a schedule 1 substance because of sound scientific proof. Surely, they must have quality reasoning as to why marijuana is in the category of the most dangerous drugs that have 'no accepted medicinal use and a high potential for abuse.'

*They didn't have the science to support that claim, and I now know that when it comes to marijuana neither of those things are true. **It doesn't have a high potential for abuse, and there are very legitimate medical applications. In fact, sometimes marijuana is the only thing that works. We have been terribly and systematically misled for nearly 70 years in the United States**, and I apologize for my own role in that."*

Aug. 8, 2013, "Why I Changed My Mind on Weed,"
CNN.com

Oct. 2003 article posted on the MDA website

THE AMERICAN NURSES ASSOCIATION (ANA):

"The American Nurses Association (ANA) recognizes that patients should have safe access to therapeutic marijuana/cannabis. **Cannabis or marijuana has been used medicinally for centuries. It has been shown to be effective in treating a wide range of symptoms and conditions.***"*

Mar. 19, 2004 "Position Statement: Providing Patients Safe Access to Therapeutic Marijuana/Cannabis," ANA website

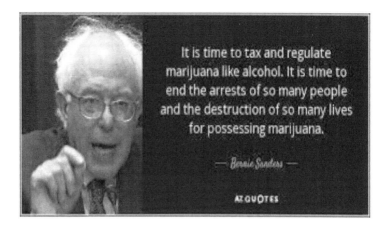

The illegality of cannabis is outrageous, an impediment to full utilization of a natural substance which helps produce the serenity and insight, sensitivity and fellowship so desperately needed in this increasingly mad and dangerous world.

Carl Sagan

Carl Edward Sagan was an American Astronomer, cosmologist, astrophysicist, astrobiologist, author, science popularizer and science communicator in astronomy and other natural sciences

Cannabis oil gives no psychoactive ("high") effect. It is pure oil that has had the THC, the psychoactive ingredient removed from it. It does however make the user more relaxed, less worried but just as productive. This is what I experienced by my use of it while it went about my body destroying cancer cells, eventually curing it. I also suffered badly from an injured shoulder—inflammation—very painful. After a short while of using the oil, I noticed that the pain had literally disappeared. There is something good about the properties of this plant. It was created by nature and when used wisely, besides healing and alleviating a myriads of illnesses, it can help bring about peace and understanding in this world that has literally gone completely insane and extremely dangerous for all its inhabitants. Can you imagine if two opposing military forces at the ready to blast each other into eternity what would happen if some good Samaritan issued to each soldier a toke of marijuana? They would simply drop their weapons and instead of slaughtering each other have a get-to-know-each-other party. It is not possible to be aggressive when using marijuana. But for the corporations, "Big Pharma" and the imperial powers, there is no profit to be made in peace. When cannabis oil is eventually approved for curing cancer and other diseases, the above, especially "Big Pharma" will stand to lose hundred of billions of dollars each year because their cancer causing drugs—chemo pills and the use of radiation will be replaced by a natural God given substance, one that the "Big Pharma" can't patent because anything from nature cannot be patented. It is all about profit and greed. It will do us well to remember each year the hundreds of thousands if not millions of people incarcerated because they did something bad under the influence of alcohol. Not one person in history has been jailed for misbehaving during the use of cannabis. A door is now opening, a door that is long overdue to help sufferers gain access to that which had been denied them for so long a time. When I was much younger, I used marijuana but once, I was not attracted to it. I liked my beer and became an alcoholic. Much later, I got cancer and found through the grapevine that cannabis oil cured cancer. I went for it. I am now cured of this wicked thing. Give it a try. It can be used along with chemo and radiation but if you have time, please try it without those chemicals; they are cancer causing and are very hard on the body and have very little success. In one hundred years the practice of treating cancer has not changed. Later, in this book, I touch on chemo and radiation's hugely negative affect on the human system. There is hope, lots of it and it is just a phone call away.

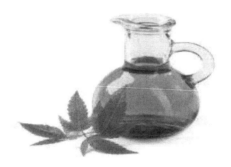

Prologue

I had heard it said many times that cancer, when diagnosed, is a death sentence. And, to be sure, in my case, that is exactly how my emotions responded. My world, as I knew it, fell apart as my mind swam in all that was death, hospitals, surgery, and chemotherapy; radiation, morticians, doctors, drugs; funeral parlors, cemeteries, cost—and the most annoying—taxes.

I remember well the words of Canada's most noble son, Terry Fox: "Cancer can happen to anyone at anytime." Well, at that time, to be sure, I thought that perhaps to others but certainly not to me. I was far removed from that kind of scourge I thought, but my ignorance and arrogance eventually caught up to me. Thirty-six years after it claimed Terry's life, it came knocking on my doorstep and, for sure, the very meaning of "death sentence" came bashing on me with its cold, sinister, terrifying onslaught. That bit of dirty news set me on a course that was to discover other approaches to dealing with, surviving and thoroughly eliminating cancer from my body. I was diagnosed with colorectal cancer and was told unequivocally that if I did not have surgery I would surely die. Even though I feared the prospects of life's finality I refused surgery and decided to give alternate natural medicines a shot. Almost two years later, I am doing fine. I gave up eating rubbish and went for organic foods along with treating my cancer directly with cannabis oil and Essiac Tea. The anti cancerous properties of these wonder plants went to work immediately diminishing my tumor until it was neutralized. These natural remedies can assist anyone in the defeat of cancer no matter the stage of the disease. Such claims are not of my accord alone, but of many, many medical and scientific professionals as well as everyday people like me.

If you have been diagnosed with cancer or have been battling it, no matter the stage, it can be reversed. You are not going to die; you are going to get very healthy and stay that way. All you have to do is follow some simple directions and you're on the way to full recovery. There are many natural cures for every disease under the sun and most certainly there are many to destroy cancer.

The following internet address is one that can benefit all persons in healing, bountiful good health, and a harmonious lifestyle. Other pertinent internet addresses are included at the end of this book.

Edgar Cayce was born March 8, 1877 on a farm close to Hopkinsville, Kentucky, USA. He was the son of a modest man who worked hard to support his family. Edgar, at an early age, had the ability to see his grandfather who had passed, and often had conversations with him. At school, Edgar had difficulty concentrating and learning. Being frustrated with his inability to concentrate, he decided to place his books beneath his pillow when he went to sleep. Upon awakening, he discovered he had the full knowledge of the contents of the book. Thus he went from last place in his school class to being the brightest student. When he left school he took a job as a photographer but a serious medical condition in his throat prevented him from speaking. All treatments proved futile. The condition lasted for over a year until one day a local hypnotist, Dr. Al Laine suggested that Edgar be put under hypnosis and see if he could diagnose his ailment. To the surprise of those in the room that day, Edgar diagnosed the problem and also prescribed the treatment for it, but not in the everyday language of the layman but in that of a learned physician. In time, following the directions for treatment, Edgar fully recovered. It was then deemed that if he could diagnose his personal ailment it could be possible to diagnose the ailments of others. The diagnosis under hypnosis was labeled "a reading". During his lifetime, Edgar Cayce gave over fourteen thousand readings; reading regarding the ailments of the individual, the cause of it and the cure for it. He also gave readings on the past, present and future of mankind and the general history of the universe. The holistic way of living was high on his advice and he was the forerunner of what we know today as holistic care and wellbeing. When Edgar Cayce awoke from his self induced trance he had no recall of what had taken place during the reading. One can only benefit from the great library of his readings that are available to all for free on the internet. More than one hundred and twenty books have been written on the universal information given to Edgar Cayce during his trance readings. One should find his works of remarkable benefit.

As the world's greatest clairvoyant, Edgar Cayce said, "In the world of plants there is a cure for very ailment and disease known to man."

edgarcayce.org

On the latter pages of this book there is information pertaining to related cancerous diseases. There are also links to videos and information that will put you on the right road to full recovery. Just get a grip on your own life and do what you must do to reverse the ailment and live a full healthful life. It is just a matter of doing it. Go on! Go for the greatest learning experience of your life!— And win! When you complete the course and cross the finish line, you will find that the

finish line is, in fact, the starting line of a full, healthy and happy life. Really! A New beginning! Go on . . . get on with it! What are you waiting for?

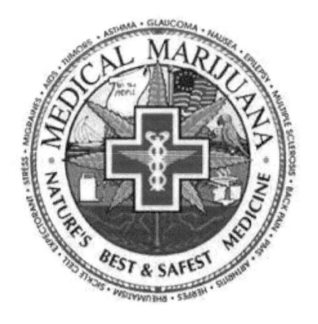

Pharmaceutical companies are interested only in profit making; that comes first; you come second—or worse—last. It is a fact. Twenty thousand people die each day from cancer; not one should have to. That translates into eight million deaths per year that are registered as cancer related, but the truth be known it is more likely twenty million. Doctors do their best with the tools that are available to them in dealing with cancer: chemo, radiation, surgery and more chemo, radiation and surgery. And as we know now, chemo and radiation are carcinogenic—cancer causing. The possibility of the cancer returning is great. And we all know that when this happens the cancer hits back with a vengeance; thus more radiation and chemo—surgery—more and more. This book is essentially about my battle with cancer, my awakening to the world of a dreadful disease, and the people who helped steer me back to a healthful life. It is a story about fear, confusion, and despondency. It is a story and it is true in every sense of the word. You can make this story yours. Just believe in the powers of the universe, the natural provisions that are available to put you right. When I was diagnosed I had little money as I always did and still have. Nevertheless, if I had been a multi-billionaire I would have gladly given every cent and borrowed if necessary to find a cure for my ailment. To me, life is sacred. I fully realized this when I was attacked by a bear when I worked in the forest. I survived that confrontation and was made realize how sacred, profound my life is and so angry that an animal had threatened to take it. That same determination to survive cancer resurfaced. This time, however, I had some time to think about my plan of survival and I got all the help I needed from people who were medical professionals who had given up on conventional treatments of cancer and with good conscience embarked on the holistic way to help victims of cancer and many other serious ailments to fully recover, people like Jesse and Chris who run the Farm Assist Medical Marijuana Outlet in Halifax, Nova Scotia, Canada. From the bottom of my heart, I thank them. Indeed, I owe them my life.

Each journey, no matter how difficult, starts with the first step. Look around and ask for assistance. There is a universe of good people ready and waiting to help. You don't have to do it alone.

Many doctors now believe that the colon is a very much neglected organ when it comes to checking for health issues and indeed it might just be the root of many if not all diseases. Just imagine if we threw some pepper and salt into each fill-up of gasoline for the car what will happen. The vehicle is not meant to deal with condiments of any kind, so too, the stomach was not engineered to deal with the multitude of preservatives and other lacings of unnatural sweeteners added to the processed foods that are in most cases the mainstream of our diets. These additives are now proven beyond doubt that they are indeed an army of silent killers made to taste palatable while they instill and plague our bodies with all kinds of diseases, one of which is cancer.

Only once did I try smoking marijuana. I never used or desired it since. I was a beer drinker and when I ran out of beer anything alcohol sufficed. I became an alcoholic. I made my life miserable and also the lives of others, especially loved ones. I lost everything that I had worked so hard for. Had I chosen cannabis,

I no doubt would have had a more productive and pleasant life.

In the 1930.s when it was discovered that the use of cannabis oil cured many illnesses, Big Pharma, with the help of corrupted government officials, including the FBI, CIA and the FDA went all out to demonize the use of Marijuana to the extreme. Now, in Canada, the country of my residency, we have a real human being running the country. He is highly intelligent, compassionate, and truly a world class leader. Under his leadership, the unfair stigma attached to marijuana has already got the boot and it will be totally de-criminalized in the days to come. This great man is beyond corruption and leads his country without the advice or interference of the politicians to the south. His name is The Honorable Justin Trudeau, Prime Minister of Canada, truly a nice bit of sunshine in the dark and dismal world of international politics.

I am not here to promote casually the use of marijuana, .but I certainly have nothing against it. If it helps people cope in a hugely stress filled world, and one increasingly dangerous, then, to be sure, I am all for it. I am primarily here to promote its healing powers and tell a truth that has long been kept in the dark. The use of cannabis oil and smoking marijuana cures and alleviates many Illness which I touch on in the following pages. But first, let us take a look at the characteristics of the oil.

Composition: Cannabis oil is a thick, guey substance, much like Black Strap Molasses, made up of cannabinoids such as THC and CBD that are extracted from the cannabis plant. Cannabis oil is a cannabis based product obtained by separating the resins from cannabis flowers, using solvents in the extraction process Cannabis oil is also know as marijuana oil, hemp oil and Phoenix Tears. The most common name used in association with the oil is **cannabis**. Cannabis oil is the most potent of three main cannabis products, which are the actual cannabis flower (marijuana), resin (hashish), and cannabis oil. Cannabis oil is the most concentrated form of the three main cannabis products. That is what makes cannabis oil the most potent.

Cannabis Oil produced and sold by back-street dealers can be contaminated and at times will have small amounts or no THC or CBD in them. Cannabis oil available on the street should be avoided for medicinal uses. It's always better to make your own oil or to have someone you trust make your oil. However, if you have obtained a medical license from your doctor, it can simply be purchased from a medical marijuana outlet. This ensures a purity and quality. High quality cannabis oil can be used in many ways medicinally and can be used for many different conditions. Cannabis Oil can be orally ingested, vaporized into the lungs, used as a suppository or applied topically.

Some conditions cannabis oil has been used for include: cancer, diabetes, Crohn's disease, gout, pain relief, glaucoma, opiod dependence, alcohol abuse, epilepsy. psoriasis, anorexia, asthma, adrenal disease, inflammatory bowel disease, fybromyalgia, rheumatoid arthritis, migraines, Dravet, Syndrome, Doose Syndrome, Multiple Sclerosis. And to further its incredible ability to cure and alleviate illnesses, Cannabis oil may also have a use as neuroprotectants for such things like limiting neurological damage following a stroke or head injury. It can also be used in the treatment of neurodegenerative diseases, such as Alzheimer's disease, Parkinson's disease and HIV dementia. It relaxes the mind promoting a more patient and clear understanding of ones' sense of well being, and when it comes to good choices, healthful food is a must for the body to recover.

Over the last several decades, the quality of our food has drastically deteriorated by the use of chemicals. Such un-nourishing stuff is extremely hard on our health, especially our colons. Our diet is the gauge that determines good health. When foods high in fats and low in fiber flood the digestive system with "stuff" that is difficult to digest the stomach is overwhelmed with sorting things out. As the body is flooded with hard-to-metabolize mass-manufactured, processed and artificial foods, the colon becomes swollen and blocked making it difficult to eliminate waste. Such "stuffing" of the body leads to a toxic buildup in the colon turning it into a storage unit for the toxic fecal matter that one struggles to eliminate.

At any given moment, the average person has up to twenty of more pounds of fecal matter inside their gut sitting there just rotting and decaying. And to make matters worse, if you suffer from Leaky Gut Syndrome this toxic fecal matter seeps through the lining of the stomach into the bloodstream—not a very nice outcome.

We live in a stressful, preservative filled, artificial ingredient world and there is a seemingly never ending list of toxins that can have and do have a negative impact on our digestive system and colon.

Everything from tap water to doctor prescribed antibiotics can and does have a negative effect on our digestive system, weakening its ability to digest. There are a variety of toxins that affect our digestive system and our colon on a daily basis, but none are more harmful than those found in our food: industrial seed oils such as corn; cottonseed, safflower, processed soybean, soy milk, soy protein; conventional dairy (non-organic) and conventional meats (non-organic). Anything processed with artificial flavors or preservatives are poisons to the system. Alcohol, too, when taken to excess is a killer of mind, body and soul. When addiction takes place life becomes a living hell.

In time, the foods and drinks mentioned above destroy our good gut bacteria, leading to an inflamed blocked colon.

It is understandable for one to rebel when it comes to shunning ones' favorite food, but one should slowly, over time, focus on those foods that are wholesomely organic. Avoid processed foods at all costs with ingredients that cannot be pronounced and stay away from bad fats and sugars. Practice moderation and make wholesomely organic decisions based on long term health, not the immediate cravings.

Two thousand years ago, Hippocrates said, "all diseases begin in the gut". Science is proving that statement correct. He is also famous for saying, "Let food be thy medicine". That statement is not an idle one.

Since the inception of Big Pharma by Rockefeller, Carnegie, J.P. Morgan and others, the Drug Lords convinced us that the holistic way of life was just sheer **"quackery"** (actually the opposite it true—Big Pharma is all about quackery) and that drugs were the way to go. Thus the wholesome way of living went into the gutter while the greedy made their billions selling all kinds of destructive "medicines". That is not to say that all drugs are a menace but the "legal" drug moguls over-did it by a long shot by closing down all naturopathic establishments that stood in competition to their multi billion dollar drug business. To this day, we see the continuing madness with the likes of genetically modified "foods" by Monsanto. All crops produced by this notorious chemical giant are not fit for consumption but such entities with their endless flow of money buy off those in power, thus the corruption is complete, and we, the people, pay for their profit making with our health—our lives.

The digestive system is an ecosystem of good and bad bacteria and research suggests that we have one hundred trillion micro-organisms *(live bacteria)* living inside our digestive tract. Good bacteria aid in digestion and elimination and bad bacteria leads to fungus, yeast infections, weight gain and serious digestive issues.

The "good bacteria" are called probiotics and are critical to a healthy digestive system. They help in the digestion of food, eliminate waste, promote healthy immune function, regulate the metabolic system and are responsible for maintaining a healthy gastrointestinal tract. A balanced digestive system is one composed of eighty percent good and twenty percent bad bacteria; when this balance is reached the digestive system functions at its best. Numerous scientific studies have proven the benefits of this healthy probiotic balance, linking probiotics to solid weight management, higher energy levels, mental clarity and a stronger immune system. It is worthwhile to remember that seventy per cent of the immune system is located in the gut.

A well balanced diet of organic food does wonders for the body: it is fuel that keeps things working constantly and properly. It promotes regularity and a sense of well being and for females it gets rid of yeast infections and other vaginal health issues that manifest due to the lack of good bacteria in the body. It promotes mental clarity and liberates the mind from anxiety, depression and negative thoughts. It gets rid of eczema, acne and other skin disorders that are a product of an unhealthy gut.

Maintaining a healthy balance of good probiotic bacteria may be the fastest, safest and easiest way to promote a healthier digestive system and colon. There are dozens of probiotics available on the market today but be sure to avoid commercially available, mass produced probiotics; they simply do not work.

To have any affect whatsoever, this sensitive bacteria needs to make it down the throat, through the stomach, past the harmful acids and into the small and large intestines. If at any point in the process they die or do not make it, taking them is completely worthless and you are literally flushing money down the drain.

Commercially produced probiotics that are sold in corporate stores like Walmart, are mass produced for cost savings and may sit in warehouses and on shelves for several months or years before being consumed. Because the live, living bacteria are very sensitive to temperature and die naturally over time, many probiotics are dead or dying before you ever take them when you buy commercially available probiotics. For this reason, it is wise to avoid off the shelf probiotics.

Make sure to purchase a probiotic supplement, from a reputable health food store. They must be probiotics produced in small batches to ensure healthy, live bacteria. Purchasing at so called money-saving outlets is taking a chance, the end result most likely being a waste of money, time and a useless product. It is your life; your health . . . be good to it. And it will make sure to beat up on negative body invaders, especially cancer.

Chapter One

My Story

Hamilton, Ontario, Canada, 2014

From my window I noticed her. She seemed almost out of place, a jogger that in every respect enjoyed each moment, each pace and breath of the run. Truly she was a person that placed her image easily upon me because I had slid into a more inactive, deskbound lifestyle. In the early days, sports, fishing, travel were all a part of my activities; however, slowly but surely

such healthy activities fell by the wayside. Indeed, I viewed the runner with a mixture of envy and admiration. Her body abounded with vigor, wellbeing and beauty, while mine slipped further into a living mess.

The mirror image set guilt upon me. I had gotten overweight by forty or more pounds. I did not like myself. Not liking me due to this condition was a good thing, because that part of my mind that acts as an irritable reminder made sure that I took stock of my bountiful blubber. No matter the angle of my body to the mirror the Sumo wrestler belly glared back at me indicating in no uncertain terms that I should get off my behind and go out and do what the runner was doing: living her life to the fullest, looking incredible healthy and making me go blue with envy. However, being generally easy-going, I attempted to put the idea of purchasing running shoes to the back in my mind in a place that would not bother me too much, but the lady runner made sure that I could not shove it too far back as to bury the health wish once and for all. She made that run each day, every day.

At that time I lived in an area known as the "Heights" in the city of Hamilton, Ontario and was making a serious attempt at writing an autobiography. My desk was set in front of my apartment window that overlooked Lake Ontario. The neighborhood was a pleasant place where many came to enjoy the view, a view that stretched across the lower city of Hamilton, on out across the massive water world of Lake Ontario. I enjoyed the view and the place but not my unhealthy condition that I tried miserably to turn a blind eye to. Music, too, was a big part of my life. I enjoyed writing compositions and also studying Spanish classical guitar; however, a shoulder injury limited my time in practice. Doctors told me that I had arthritis in the shoulder and that it would only get worse and that the best thing to do was to take anti-inflammatory pills to lessen the pain. Still, I did not like taking such pills as they nauseated my stomach and made me irritable. One day, however, the pain was severe and I decided to visit the doctor.

And she was a doctor, a very thorough and dedicated doctor. It was the first time that I had met Dr. Ing. She informed me that to have the anti-inflammatory medicine she would have to take my blood pressure because if the pressure is high the pills can cause some health issues.

That was the beginning of information that was all bad—very, very bad. I was informed that my blood-pressure was dangerously high and that she had to make some more tests.

When all was said and done, I was borderline diabetic and had an irregular heartbeat—arrhythmia, along with cholesterol build-up and a host of other things that made for a very unhealthy overweight body. Dr. Ing did not miss that belly bulge. When she had concluded the tests she told me that I had an eighty percent chance of stroke or heart attack—maybe both. She then backed handed me on the belly and told me to go lose that which was killing me slowly. I listened. That particular day was in late autumn of 2014. I purchased the running shoes, put them on and went jogging. I had just being gifted with a mighty wake-up call. I was happy that the sidewalk was absent of sports-minded people. I was embarrassed with my pace of run. Nevertheless, I went for it and gave it my best. Next, I decided to lose all that weight in a few weeks. I went on the master-cleanse, a body cleansing called The Bragg Master Cleanse, a cleansing with pure lemon juice, water, maple syrup and a dash of cayenne pepper. That is all I consumed for sixteen days—no solid food of any kind—just the drink. I did lose that weight.

After more tests, I was sent to see a heart specialist. I was informed that my heart was very strong but the irregular beat was something of a mystery and that more tests might reveal the problem. Still, I kept on jogging and did lots of walking. With the great "belly bulge" gone I began to feel better; nevertheless, my doctor did not prescribe the anti-inflammatory pills. I eventually put up with the pain and forgot about attempting to obtain them.

The physical exercises continued. The runner, whom I eventually named "Princess", continued her clockwork routine. It was, to be sure, something she enjoyed. She looked the picture of bountiful health and she exuded everything that pertained to naturalness, beauty and ultimate wellbeing. She would never know it but she would bring about the spark that would catapult me back into the world of nutritious living—at least for a while. I continued to jog and to eat less unhealthy foods. My blood pressure normalized and the diabetes and cholesterol lessened. Just doing those simple but challenging steps I had reduced myself of three potential killers, but not all was gravy; the problem with my heart could not be determined. I accepted the unqualified verdict and upped my jog to a bit of sprinting—not bad for a fellow in his sixty-eight year. Still, Dr. Ing had not finished with me. She was relentless in pursuing those things that might be wrong with me.

Indeed, she was born to be a doctor, a caring, intelligent, devoted doctor. She had chosen her line of work to perfection. I developed a great respect for her. The tests revealed that my blood count was out of whack but what was causing it was another matter. Eventually, I had a fecal test. Weeks later, I got a call from the clinic. I was asked to make an appointment to see the doctor but that it was not an emergency. Those words, "not an emergency", gave me much comfort. I had decided to move from Ontario to Nova Scotia for the purpose of promoting my literary works; however, that decision was to have unforeseen, dire consequences, but consequences that would steer me in a direction that would unveil the world of cancer and its unrelenting plague.

It Takes Only One Person

To Change Your Life—You!

Chapter Two

Death Sentence

Some months later after my arrival in Nova Scotia, I noticed a blood discharge when I had a bowel movement. But, being me, I made all kind of excuses about it being "nothing serious". The truth is that I was afraid it was something serious and hoped that it would clear up. It didn't. It persisted to the point that forced me to see the doctor. I was asked if my family had a history of colon cancer to which I replied that I did not know. Nevertheless, that word "cancer" made me uneasy—scared. I was hoping that it was something less severe and that a pill or two would fix it. I was informed that an appointment would be made to see the oncologist and that I would be contacted when a date was set. Three weeks had passed. I had not heard back from the oncologist's office in regards to my appointment. I grew concerned and phoned the doctor's office. It is also important that when making an appointment that it is understood that the system is not perfect and one can run into the unexpected, the unexpected that bring about more anxiety. People who work within the system, while not being uncompassionate, can become removed or complacent to one's disposition. Of course, such behavior can stem from being in a hugely negative environment, where each day, the medical personal are dealing with ill people, and indeed that might well bring about a casual response, seemingly void of concern. Perhaps it is a defensive mechanism. Such casualness is what I experienced all throughout the medical system. Please be prepared for such encounters. I truly felt that I was embarking on a mission impossible through a very huge factory. The initial contact is summed up as follows when I made that phone call:

Oh, said the receptionist, it can take up to many months before you get to see an oncologist."

I understand that a long wait to see a specialist in the medical system is standard but that was not my question. I wanted to know if an appointment had been made for me. "I understand that," I replied, "but it should take at the most a couple of days to make the appointment."

The irritating senselessness continued "Oh, but you see it is summer time and the oncologist is away on vacation."

I am usually an easygoing person and quickly disassociate from dumb conversations but this one was a life and death one. I raised my voice. "For heavens sake, I will be dead and buried before I get any kind of medical treatment at this rate . . . is there just one oncologist operating in the city"?

"Well, there are others but they have to take up the slack when one is off on vacation." She continued. "It might be more to your benefit if call the oncologist's office and see where you are on the list. I will give you the number and you can get in touch with them. Maybe it will speed things up."

Out of sheer frustration, I kept my mouth closed and accepted the phone number, but the frustration continued with an answering device "Thank you for the call. This office does not return calls. Please go through your doctor's office for information regarding your appointment."

Again, I could hardly believe my ears. However, I did leave a message just in case on the "off chance" that someone might listen to my "call on the wind". It seemed to work. Within the following two weeks I received confirmation of the appointment. It was all nerve-racking stuff. Like all people, I suppose, that await the sentence, a sentence that might be terminal, semi terminal, or lesser. I was worried—very worried. After the colon inspection, I was curtly told that I had cancer and that I needed surgery. Those words shivered cold through my blood. I went into a state of shock. And while I was falling apart the oncologist said that he would make an appointment for me to see the radiologist and the surgeon.

Indeed, upon receiving such debilitating news my world turned upside down. Where to go and what to do was all consuming because I had no idea as to where to go or what to do; my life now was totally in the hands of others. On the way home from the medical clinic, I walked the short-cut, which I usually did, along the railroad tracks that run by my home and got lost in the kicking my mind and body just received. After all, I just found out that I am a mortal and that I am going to die. On the rail I sat, lost in the devastating immensity of life's looming finality. I wanted to cry more than anytime I could remember, but the tears would not come.

Suddenly, all those things I thought were important were not important. All that I thought I had accomplished was not important and just as unimportant were all those things that I had felt guilty about. They, too, were given a break. The only thing that seemed of any importance to me was the fact that I was alive and that I had cancer and that I had to do something about it but what that might be I had no idea. My mind just swam in the fogginess and echoes of the words, **CHEMO and RADIATION.** It was something that I thought could and would never happen to me. Well, it did happen to me. My life, as I knew it, came to a crashing halt. It was replaced with the fear of the unknown—the dark and dismal dimensions of cancer. That was it. I went off to await the further processes of my treatments. I waited for that phone call. Two weeks passed and still no word.

Eventually, a call came from my oncologist. He wanted to see me. Again the worrying set in. I knew now for sure what is meant by the old adage: *When you have your health you have everything.*

When I went to see the oncologist he asked if I had seen the surgeon and radiologist. I told him that I had not, that I was still waiting. I could see that he was upset as the lackadaisical attitude and told me that he would speed things up. It was obvious that he was concerned at the rate my cancer was spreading, and to be sure, so was I. He told me that he would speed things up, and true to his word, he did. Within two days I was off the see the hospital team.

I began to notice that being accepted into proper care that it takes a long time because the system is absolutely overloaded. It does its best but falls short by a long shot, be that as it may. If you do not have private medical insurance and have to go through the public system, be prepared for the waits. It is just that way

After the catscan was taken I was sent off again into the murky grey world of waiting. And to be sure it is grey and very bleak. The result of the catscan was not encouraging. The cancer was mustering its troops for the big siege and plunder of the rest of my body. It had spread into the prostrate gland and into the stomach. It was all bad. Nevertheless, I again decided to go on "The Master Cleanse". The decision put me in a more positive frame of mind; being proactive in my healing helped release the constant worry that consumed my every moment.

After the catscan, I was sent to see the surgeon and her assistant. I was told the usual stuff—stuff that seems to have no explanation and no reassurance attached to it. It was all pleasant enough chat with everyone hoping for the best. The medical staff did their best to relax me about the nasty characteristics of the disease and its treatments. Still, we were all aware that cancer had a big unpleasant mind of its own and killing people was its thing—it's only thing. Now it was preparing to do me in. Slowly but surely the killer was beginning to tear my insides apart and rebuild it to its own murdering specifications. And the news got worse, a lot worse.

"There is a possibility that you will be **rendered impotent,"** said the radiologist. "The cancer is very close to the prostrate gland." He went on. "There is not much we can do about that; it's just the way cancer operates."

And while the Radiologist carried on informing me of the many things that could, would, might, and maybe go wrong my mind blazed about the second cataclysmic bit of news that was so casually imparted to me—**the coming of my impotence.** There was no reining in my emotional tremor. What I had heard was the nuclear explosion of shock waves saturating my body, mind, and spirit. The cancer killing me was bad news but not as bad as the coming of my "impotence", a word that caused to me some confusion.

"Do you mean that the radiation treatments will make me sexually dysfunctional?"

"Oh, in such cases," said the Radiologist, rather smugly, "one can always purchase the sexual activation pills. You can always take one and it will help in such matters." I was not impressed. Along with a prescription for chemo pills, anti-nauseous and anti-diarrhea pills, the bad news continued as a **yellow card** was presented to me. "If you pass out or are feeling bad . . . high blood pressure, racing heart, heart attack, hot and cold sweats; shortness of breath, diarrhea, yellow jaundice, impaired vision . . . just take this card with you to emergency; it will help open the door to treatment a bit faster." The negative forecast went on. "Oh, and for sure you will break out in sores on your mouth and the lower extremities of your body but they should clear up over time, if not we can prescribe a drug to help."

I thought, *always a drug to help, a drug to counteract the damage of its counterpart.* To be sure, there was not one measure of positive news associated with the remedial procedures. I just listened in stunned silence as one might to a judge who had placed the black cap on his head before handing down the death sentence. I lived alone. I wondered how I was going to get to emergency if I had a heart attack and, for sure, I understood what it was like to have one foot on a banana peel and the other in a grave. Indeed, the face of death was but smiling over me. I would just have to absorb as bravely as I could the bad, sad news. The Radiologist went on. "You are in excellent shape. You are not presently on any medication. This should help you enormously in your battle."

I did not want to hear any more. My body sagged and my mind went soggy; I was a mess. Off I went with my **"yellow card"** into a world of continued shock and confusion. But the facts of my illness were in my face. There could be no more denial—no more pretending. I had to find the will and the courage to take on this tyrant and defeat it.

It was just some months before my seventieth birthday when I got the sentence. I have lived alone for many years. I was free to go anywhere I wished as long as I could afford it. But now, things suddenly changed and, to be sure, not for the better. I was a captive of cancer. My mind swam in the desperate emptiness as death's finger pointed unwaveringly at me.

The twenty-seven treatments of **Chemo and radiation** made me feel tired, sick, and irritable. I had been a smoker. I smoked one to two packs of cigarettes a day for many years. I also drank alcohol for many years. I was addicted to both. Alcohol was the first to go. It had taken a good twenty years of my life and all the money I worked hard for before it released me. That was a tough one but I managed to quit. Some years later, I brought the cigarette habit to an end. However, as the radiologist predicted, the sore and scabs manifested and made my life more miserable. My lips looked like I had been in the boxing ring with Mohamed Ali and he just used my mouth as a punching bag. They were largely swollen and took on a fractured, raw, deep glistening purplish color. My lower extremities suffered the same. I was just happy that my eyes were not positioned to view them and the last thing I intended to do was use a mirror. It was all very unappealing looking at a body disintegrating in a mess of scabs. And, to be sure, if that was the way I had to live then for sure I would wish a speedy exit from my earthly home. In time, however, the unwanted disappeared only to be replaced by something equally unappealing but with a horrid, painful, fiery sensation—radiation burn. And that extremely unpleasant experience I was not informed about.

Approximately a month after the radiation treatments, I felt an intense burning sensation throughout my colon. I had no idea as to what it was but it felt like I was sitting on a hot stove. It was painfully uncomfortable and caused me great irritation. My family doctor was away on vacation so I went to see a doctor at a walk-in clinic. He figured that it might be *H-Pylori*, a parasite that dwells in the stomachs of most of the world's population. A blood test was taken and it was positive. I was elated because I felt that it was cancer that was causing the problem.

Drugs were prescribed to deal a mortal blow to the unwanted stomach dweller but no relief came. Later, at a meeting with my surgeon, I was told that it was the radiation, that is was just one of those many side effects. That part of the trip was extremely painful and worrisome and I was much annoyed that I had not been foretold of this other "side effect". To be sure, I was getting a very good apprenticeship in the massive negative methodology of dealing with the curse of cancer and all the while I lived in the clutches of a monster that was adverse to kindness and mercy.

Only I Can Change My Life

No One Can Do It For Me

Chapter Three

The Search

There is a weekend farmers' market at the Alderney Landing in Dartmouth, Nova Scotia. I went there occasionally to purchase organic fresh veggies and at times rented a table and displayed my books. It was during that time I met Ben, a designer and trader in leather goods. It was this man that set me on course to find alternative cures for cancer. Indeed, he was a Godsend. He directed me to *Chrisbeatcancer.com,* and that information *was* a Godsend. Ten years before Chris had exactly what I was dealing with—stage three colon cancer that was quickly moving toward stage four. However, Chris was whisked almost immediately into the operating room for surgery. After the operation he was told that he would need up to a year or more of chemo and radiation. That heavy bombardment of treatment he clearly refused even though medical professionals, family and friends pressured him to do so. Still, he did not relent. He was aware of the carcinogenic (cancer causing) properties of radiation and chemo; I was not. Ten years later, Chris is alive and in perfect health. I was impressed with his presentation and knowledge of the cancer-world and the holistic approach in dealing with it. Organic fresh vegetables, leafy greens, vegetable juice, and most particularly carrot juice were part of his offensive armor in striking back against the wicked invader. After listening to one of his many videos, I immediately tossed out all processed foods from my diet and went for only organic foods. Ben, also put me onto the use of cannabis oil in the treatment of cancer. That very surprising bit of information perked my ears, but where to find a source for the oil was to be challenging. It would take a bit of time, but I intuitively believed I was onto something that would prove its worth in beating cancer and, whatever it took, I was going to avail myself of it. To be sure, it was truly a formidable search. But as fate had it, a room mate used a toke marijuana more than occasionally. Still, I was in a bit of an embarrassing bind because I had given him a piece of my mind a few months earlier for smoking the stuff in the house. He apologized. Now, with tongue in cheek, I mustered the courage and asked him where I might avail that which might save my life marijuana. To my surprise, he had a network of contacts that supplied him with that which eased his worldly concerns, but the one that most garnered my attention was a place called Farm Assist, a medical marijuana outlet on Gottengen St., in the city of Halifax that supplied all forms of cannabis products to people who, in their last resort, found relief from their physical and mental trials. How quickly I put aside my condemnation of those, who over the many years, I had silently rebuked for the use of such a waste-making substance; how quickly I was made aware of my hypocrisy. Now, swallowing my useless pride, I made a visit to the dispensary on Gottengen Street. There I was told that I would have to acquire from my family doctor a medical marijuana license in order to obtain the oil. With the stigma and prejudice toward cannabis use permeating the medical system, I was back to square one in my search. But such obstacles only served to intensify my quest for that which gave hope in curing my cancer. I did not need any prompting to see my family doctor. Still, I had reservations as to his mind-set in regards to the use of marijuana. Many doctors hold a negative view of the use of marijuana. Drugs are what they are trained to necessitate. However, to my surprise, he was fully aware of marijuana's potential treatment for cancer and of many other illnesse. Nevertheless, he could not issue a license to me because he was not adept in the medical know-how of cannabis but instantly referred me to a government medical representative. At last, I was on the right path but disappointment hit me almost immediately—there was a two month waiting period to see the medical marijuana doctor. However, a couple of days later, I received a phone call from the medical license cannabis center and was told that I could see the doctor the following day. I was elated. A first time fee of one hundred dollars was paid then my license was approved; it was good for a twelve month period.

I immediately phoned a marijuana government approved outlet that was located in New Brunswick. The outlet on Gottengen Street had not been government approved. It at times had been raided by the police, but never closed down—leave that to one's imagination.

The New Brunswick dispensary informed me that they did not have the cannabis oil in stock but that I could make the oil. All I had to do was follow the directions. I paid close to three hundred dollars for one ounce. When I received the packet by mail I immediately set about making the oil. To process it, I needed a small rice cooker and a bottle of one hundred percent ethyl alcohol, a product available at most pharmacies. I placed the contents of the packet into the cooker, poured the full bottle of alcohol over it and let it simmer until the ethyl alcohol had evaporated. Not been aware of the outcome of the processing, I used the facilities of the kitchen and not long into the operation, I was hit with an odor that was so much stronger than that of what I had experienced when my room mate toked in the house. I immediately panicked and took the electric cooker outside the house but the smell only intensified and permeated the neighborhood. How embarrassed I was; nevertheless, I completed the process and was quiet disappointed with the tiny amount of oil extracted. It looked so dismal, but I did not realize the powerful punch that occupied that miserable looking bit of gluey goo. Since the time I had been diagnosed with cancer I had become dispirited. I had never taken any kind of drugs to ward off bad times. Now, however, I needed help. A couple of weeks before, from the doctor, I got a prescription for some drug or other to deal with my anxiety. The drug did, to a good extent, relieve my bothersome mind. I was able to navigate almost a normal daily routine. But that all changed when I ingested the cannabis oil, an amount equal to that of a small grain of rice.

How long I had passed out I do not know, but when I regained consciousness, I had no idea as to who I was or where I was. My mind seemed to hang somewhere in eternity with no sense of direction other than it was a mind and one that was very lost. I felt that I had had a stroke or a heart attack, even both. I just sat in a chair with my eyes glued to the computer monitor. As minutes passed, I became more afraid than I had ever been in my entire life: my identity, as I knew it, was gone. Just thinking about the prospect of getting to my bed, which was just inches away, presented an unbelievable effort, but I had to attempt it. If I failed, then I would end up crashing on the floor; but I did make it—barely. As I lay on my back, looking to the ceiling, much like the first time that I had over indulged in alcohol, my head spun and my stomach churned. To get to the hospital was my immediate goal; but I could not stand; neither could I make a phone call; my normal physical abilities had vanished as the feeling of total helplessness set in. I was afraid, very afraid.

With each passing moment, my inner senses prompted me to arise and make every effort to get to the hospital, but truly, I was in no shape to be going anywhere, not even to the cemetery. Still, I had to muster whatever was left of me to arise from the bed and seek help, but from whom? The only source of local help, my house mate, was off on vacation. Still, I was somewhat alive and although my situation seemed hopeless, from the deepest part of my soul came the call to do the almost impossible—to get off the bed and no matter my condition to get out of the house and point myself towards the hospital. That I did with great difficulty. Just to make it to sitting on the side of the bed was incredibly challenging, but I did make it. At that point, I realized that I had lost my ability to speak and even to think clearly, but I had to get to the hospital. With every difficulty, I stood, balancing as best I could, but the sensation was that of standing on a two legged stool with a rope around my neck. Then I thought that if I attempted to walk that effort might give me the desired balance, but it didn't; I fell heavily on the floor. Again, I picked myself up and again with greater determination I managed to grab a jacket and struggle it on. The same mind-boggling procedure went with putting my shoes and socks on. Eventually, I grabbed my "yellow card" and truly felt some relief that it was in my hand because if I got lost or fell over, those who found me would have some idea as to what I was about. Thus began the longest, most torturous journey of my life in a body that felt it was scattered all over the universe.

Along the pavement I stumbled and crumbled, but I kept going with a mind outside my body prompting me onwards, but in truth I was terrified that the man I knew was no more and that I had been replaced by something detached of reason, compassion, understanding—all sense of self. Still, on I went in my sway-like motions, praying incessantly, just like that first time I had flown across the English Channel in a twin engine aircraft: the rattling, shaking, dipping and swaying; the cutlery bouncing noisily on the food trays, the air hostess lacking the ability to hide her fear as she buckled her safety strap. And now, fifty years later, all that fear returned, but magnified to a great degree. Eventually, what appeared to be an ice-chilling midnight stumble through desolations' matrix, the light that I craved appeared— the hospital's emergency entrance. I at last made it to the door of hope. Out of the wind-jeering night and into the welcoming light of the emergency room, with "yellow card" in hand, I arrived. There, I swayed like a plant might in a gentle breeze as I awaited my turn to register and present my "yellow card". I was asked about my problem, but I could not speak. I was handed back my "yellow card" and curtly told to take a place in the line-up and wait for assessment—so much for my "yellow card" speeding up things. Eventually, I got to see the processor. By that time, I was able to utter almost inaudibly as to my situation. Tests were done to determine if I were diabetic, an illness that had been determined by Dr, Ing as borderline, back in Hamilton, a couple of years prior. The tests concluded all was normal. I was not diabetic and my blood pressure was normal. Nevertheless, I was asked to take a seat and await the doctor's prognosis. At this point, slowly, very slowly I began to regain some semblance of my former self but I still could not stand with any confidence. I even practiced speaking, but it was still just utters accompanied by mutters, stutters and despondency. Eventually, after an hour or so, the doctor appeared. My voice had to some degree improved. I was able to explain, as far as I could remember, that I had taken cannabis oil along with some 'yellow pill', an anti anxiety drug, and since then my body, soul and spirit seemed to have deserted me.

She nodded and smiled. "Yes, that will do it," she said, "but I am going to admit you just to make sure."

She was a nice person. I felt comfortable with her. The following morning I was awakened by a doctor who had just come on shift. "You are all ready to go home," he said. "Cannabis oil for cancer is ok in my books, especially with what you have. Just make sure you use the highest quality. Some of that stuff is questionable; make sure you get it from a reputable supplier."

I did not know it at the time but that doctor was one with an open mind and one that understood the benefits of cannabis oil. Big Pharma did not own him.

With those words, he released me from hospital care and sent me on my way. My voice had returned, and with it my mind, body, and spirit. I was so thankful just to me no matter my perceived difficulties. Before the radiation and chemo treatments commenced, I was told not to take certain medications nor was I to partake of alternative natural herbal remedies. When I informed the surgeon's assistant about my interest in cannabis oil, I was advised not to take it for at least two weeks after the treatments commenced. I did not ask for the reasons because I am not that much of a curious fellow, but my mind did entertain mildly as to why? Not long after, I got to understand fully the reason I was given that directive.

During the days following, I began to notice the lessening of rectal bleeding. In a couple of weeks, the bleeding had completely subsided. Later, much later, it dawned on me that the reason of the request not to take cannabis-oil, and other anti cancer combatants at the initial stages of chemo and radiation treatment was that the medical establishment was very much aware that cannabis-oil did the same thing, but at that time I did not know that.

The process of making cannabis oil, for me, proved difficult and costly. I did not have a private place where I could conduct the process. I again approached the outlet, Farm Assist, on

Gottengen Street. I was received warmly and offered as much help as I needed. It was at Farm Assist that I truly saw first hand the suffering of the many: people who had unsuccessful surgery, and not just with cancer but a wide variety of chronic ailments including epilepsy, asthma, fibromyalgia, depression, back aches, stomach ulcers, IBS, Crohn's Disease . . . on and on. The pharmaceutical drugs prescribed, in most cases, only made matters worse for the sufferer. It was truly there that I observed the miracle in the healing power of the marijuana plant. The plant, as its use in recorded history, is as old as man but perhaps billions of years in its evolution.

Eventually, the twenty-seven sessions of radiation along with the ingesting of four chemo pills prior to radiation were completed. I felt relieved. I could now concentrate on other commitments until a follow-up appointment for an additional catscan. I was informed that the tumor had shrunk to that size suitable for surgical removal. I was relieved about the results but my inner voice demanded me to avoid surgery. When I aired my views, a bewildering look beset both the surgeon and the interns who accompanied her. Apparently, from what I observed, the words I had uttered were beyond unusual. The disbelief exhibited on the faces of those present indicated that along with my cancer I also had a major mental illness. That, I don't dispute, but for sure, no surgeon's scalpel was going to cut into my flesh in regards to my cancer, that I was unequivocally determined about. Eventually, the surgeon suggested that I have a sigmioscopy—a lesser form of a colonoscopy—a procedure where a camera is inserted into the colon to view the tumor. Indeed, it was out of concern for my very life that she suggested the procedure and I complied. I was aware that the doctor had my best interests at heart. I respected her. Almost immediately, I was sent to have the inspection. During the inspection, I was allowed to view the procedure on the monitor. I was relatively calm in a bubble of heightened apprehension as the camera coursed its way through the colon. The "ahahs" of the oncologist seemed to carry a positive tone while he directed the camera lens and what I was hoping for appeared throughout my colon—the absence of anything that looked like a tumor. Still, I kept my mouth shut and hoped for the best. At that point, the doctor asked his assistant to call the surgeon and have her come to view the results. Truly, I did not know what to expect, but when the surgeon arrived and made the inspection she smiled and obliged me to have an MRI to determine the presence or absence of cancer in other areas of my body. The oncologist, too, nodded his head and said it was all looking good. I was elated, but still not free. A few days later the results of the MRI showed that the cancer was clear of the prostrate gland and the stomach, but there was a concern about the slight remainder of the tumor. I was told again that I must have surgery but my instincts ran contrary to such advice. This inner advice was not of imagination. Years before, when I was a forest worker, I had an experience that left no doubt about a force within, a connection to the "other world", the unseen entities that are constantly with us; those who have gone before us—those who love and protect us. To be sure, I needed their help from time to time, actually, all the time, to be truthful.

Akin to a snow covered narrow bridge, across the banks of a frozen stream rested a gigantic snow-clad tree. Removing a short handle shovel from my pack, I began the routine procedure of snow clearing. An hour's shoveling exposed the tree's thick bark. It was a cedar tree, the wood which I sought. Climbing to the topside of the tree with chainsaw in hand, I edged across to its centre and there made a test-cut. Dcep, rich, red chips spit out with the saws bite. I was not disappointed. The wood was solid, such a find helping to ease the disappointments of the day. However, with darkness descending, it was time to leave the forest.

Early morning light gave proof to the night's intense snowfall. The red ribbon marker I had hung in a tree branch the previous day indicated my work area where the tools lay beneath the snow. Three hours of snow clearing saw the tree uncovered. It was time to dissect the great cedar. However, it is said that no matter the experience of the forest worker, the unexpected, or carelessness can, in the twinkling of an eye, unhinge the plans.

The wind was at ease as I primed my saw and made ready to dissect the tree, but there was an unease gathering in me. Something was amiss, but of its nature I was unaware. Closing my mind to the unsettling thoughts, I set about my work and with chainsaw in hand I crouched beneath the great cedar at its center point and began to cut upwards. It was an unfathomable mistake. As the saw spit out the wood chips a voice raged through my mind that I was in serious danger and to stop cutting and get out from under the tree. I ignored the voice. I should have listened. I had forgotten that I had made a test cut on the top of the tree the previous evening. The tree instantly collapsed on top of me. I remember my words: "It is over; I am dead".

I had no idea how much time had passed but I found myself looking back from a hillside at the collapsed tree. I was unsure if I had been killed but I was not afraid. I was aware that someone was with me, someone I could not see. I pinched myself hard to feel for feeling and all seemed o.k. but I was still unsure of which dimension I existed in. Calmly I sat in the silk-white snow, my snowshoes still strapped to my feet, my body still clad in my heavy winter attire, my tools still strapped around my waist, my eyes glued to where the tree had collapsed at the halfway point. It just lay there broken like two gigantic shafts reaching in from the stream's banks angling down to meet each other at the center point of the frozen stream, my chainsaw and axe trapped beneath and, maybe me, too. Had I been crushed? That was the question. I could feel or see no reason why my body was not under the tree and I believed that surely it was. Yet, my eyes were drawn to a particular spot of light that seemed to hang just above the snow covered ground, an orb of light; a spot of shining comfort just there in front of me as though it were smiling at me. And I smiled back in wonder of what had taken place. Still, I was not sure if I was in spirit form or that of the flesh. The question was if someone would come and guide me through the unfamiliar dimensions. Perhaps I had to figure it out for myself. Still, the orb of light remained and I felt unthreatened as a great hush fell across the woodlands, a pure and surreal quietness that I hitherto had not experienced except for my out of body travels. Then, to jump into the sheer tranquility as though it were created for the furry martin, a cousin to the otter and ferret, the petite creature skipped and hopped across the virgin snow as though the curtains were pulled and the theater of nature was all about him. It was an astonishing moment leaving me to think that this extraordinary place of natural beauty was created just for the martin and that I was an intruder. I watched as he enjoyed his world, the odd conifer branch unloading its icy-snow burden, flicking its frozen load to the powder snow below and bounce back to its natural lay while in the distance the massive ice sheets of the mighty Columbia River echoed its thunder across the valley as the ice split in its natural flow and force. Indeed, it was a cold, cold world of snow bound beauty and I was still wondering if I had been killed.

Eventually, I got to my feet and focusing on the center point of the collapsed tree, I walked slowly down the hillside, counting my strides as I went, my eyes still glued to that part where under lay my axe and chainsaw, and maybe me—I was looking for my body. A deep sadness pressed itself upon me as I thought about the ending of my life: *Had I traveled and experienced so much in the world to have my life end in the Canadian forest?* Still, as I edged closer to the point of reckoning, I warily sought out my body—an arm—a leg showing from beneath the tree but they were not to be seen other than what was attached to my walking body. How strange those moments, and those moments continued, especially when working in the forest.

I shudder when I think back to that particular day. And I always ask the question: *did I die out there in the forest? Am I really in this dimension that I think I am thinking in?* And, to be truthful, I am not sure. There is so much more to our existence than meets the eye. And the question remains: how on earth did I end up on a hill forty feet away from where the tree collapsed? Just how did I get there? Did I have some unknown flying talent that I was unaware of that caused me to fly to a safe space on the side of a hill? Even the greatest long distance jumpers in the world would have reached only half that distance—if that. No, I did not have a pilot's license to fly at will across the land, and the only flying I ever did under my own design was that of falling out of a tree—many times. And what about the orb of bright light; what and who was that? Was that my saving grace? Was that orb some good spirit—an angel who lifted me from danger and placed me in safety? That, surely, is the only rational answer that can be presented in this case; but, then again, I might ask—*why me?*

As I left the forest that day, I stopped briefly to view the spectacular scenery that was part of the Columbia valley; it was stunning, majestic, beautiful. And as I set my eyes across the snow clad land the world before me seemed to meld into one natural energy, that of the sky and the earth and all that was in the earth appeared to be one constant flow of inseparable energy which possessed a consciousness of complete harmony and peace—no shifts in emotions, just a peaceful flow of consciousness like that of an untroubled meandering stream. In that place all was harmonized peace, a place that knew not a trouble or unsettling thoughts. So natural it was that time and space did not exist. It just was. And while there, the bothersome things of my world were non existent; I was part of a consciousness, a perfect blend of all that was good. And as I lingered in that state of spiritual perfection, I was fully aware of my duel existence, a mirror me existing simultaneously in two dimensions and it all appeared and felt perfectly natural. Those were moments that I wished would continue forever—that of perfect harmony—all with one and one with all.

The voice from within that told me to get out from under the tree was the same that told me not to have the surgery and, to be sure, I listened. I had heard of the many complications associated with such procedures, the continuing drug treatment, more complications and more surgery, the crippling of the body and the painful, slow deaths—deaths that were delayed, but inevitable.

If I were to die then I just wanted to go as soon as possible and get it over with. I was beginning to accept my finality, a finality that was attached to dignity and as little pain as possible, and not to be alone, especially not being alone when I moved on.

A few days later, I received a call from my family doctor. I was requested to see him. He read that which had been emailed to him from my surgeon: *'if I did not have the surgery it was certain that I would die'*. Again, I went foggy and numb and was relieved just to get out of the doctor's office. Walking, for me, was therapeutic. It relieved my anxiety to a large degree, and sometimes I walked until I could no more. And, to be sure, when I was given by my family doctor the certainty of my death, I did a lot of walking and determined with more resolve not to have the surgery. I would await the results of the MRI. Being free from medical procedures was like a wonderful breath of springtime fresh air, a warm and gentle sun giving pleasantness across my mind. They were the days that I savored, like a well deserved cool drink after a hard days work. But as the dreaded visit drew closer I became unsettled and tried hard to clear it from my mind, but the little devils were there constantly reminding me of my mortality as time moved inexorably towards the moment of truth. How I dreaded such moments, moments filled with fear and uncertainty—the long anxious walk filled with fear and dread, a walk that I had to complete and at its end wait nervously for the surgeon to impart the results of the MRI. Those moments awaiting the news were the worst. I had run out of spring-time-sun moments as the great cloud of darkness descended and engulfed what appeared to be a very tiny man—me. Still, I was a man no matter how diminished or fear ridden I was, no matter the weariness of my shallow breathing, I was still alive. But the question that truly pummeled the moment was for how long would I be breathing? Truly, they were horrible moments and for certain I now knew the inner suffering of those in the same quagmire of existence: pain, despondency, helplessness. Eventually it was explained that the tumor had lessened significantly but there was still concern. Instantly my heart warmed and elated beads of light danced randomly through my head. I was now convinced that the cannabis oil was doing its job but kept my thoughts to myself. The surgeon went on. "It is a good time to do surgery, I think you should really consider."

I replied that I would rather continue using the cannabis oil and that I was afraid of the results of the operation to which she replied that at times it is successful and there is nothing to fear. But I was in fear and asked that question that might decide if I should comply—the chances of my having to wear a colostomy bag. It was a direct question and received a direct answer. I was told that in my case the chances were fifty-fifty. Those stats did not sit well with me. Only if my death were imminent would I even consider such a venture. To my surprise, I was told that my decision was understandable, that the complications given to such surgery can lead to a very painful death and if "complications" set in, a common word in medical procedures, the crippling of the body begins followed by more drugs and more surgery—that it was not a nice way to die. I needed to hear what was said and it was said without reservation. After some more discussion it was suggested that "we wait and see" . . . that in two more months a catscan should be taken and await the results. And that is what happened. The results showed that the tumor was now benign, just lazing there as lifeless as a dead mouse, but that is not what I was told by the intern who preceded the surgeon with questions, which was usually the case. I was told by her that pretty much what I had been told at the previous meeting: that there was a lessening of the tumor and that it was a good time to have the surgery. I became guarded. I asked her what the chances of successful surgery were and also what the chances of not having to wear a colostomy bag. I was told that it was a hundred percent certain that I would have to wear the bag. I replied that I did not intend to have the surgery, that I would continue to use the cannabis oil and also a tea that is renowned for curing cancer—Essiac Tea, a tea that had come to my attention a few days before. She heard of neither in the use of healing cancer. She then left the room and told me she would be back in a few minutes with the surgeon. Again, I waited in uncertainty but resolved not to have surgery. When the surgeon appeared she told a completely different story. She said that all areas of the body were clear and that the tumor had been neutralized—it was dormant—a tiny lobe sitting around doing nothing. She then smiled and said, "I guess you are one of the two percent that chemo and radiation has worked for."

Out of respect I kept my mouth shut, but truly, in my heart I knew that it was the cannabis oil and the Essiac Tea, plus the organic way of eating that had truly worked. It was suggested that a six month period should pass before I received the next catscan. But to be truthful, I did not want to see the inside of a hospital again and I went literally on my merry way. I did not return. I knew in my heart that my cancer was eliminated—that I was now free, and that I had found another great friend that is renowned for curing cancer—Essiac Tea.

Nevertheless, to this day, I can't figure why the intern told me a different story as to that of the surgeon. Perhaps she had read an earlier report on my medical situation, but no matter the cause, it could well have been disastrous for me if I had not been asking the right questions, believing in the cure of cannabis oil, and being mentally prepared for the highly charged negative approach towards the treatment of cancer by medical personnel and friends alike. Christopher Wark of Crissbeatcancer.com had done his job to perfection.

A Healthy Lifestyle

Not Only Changes Your Body

It Changes Your Mind

Your Attitude And Your Mood

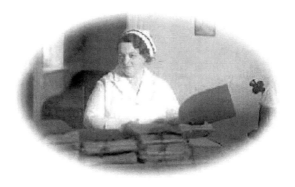

Nurse Rene Caisse, circa 1930

Chapter Four

Essiac Tea and Nurse Rene Caisse

Quote From Nurse Rene Caisse

"From 1934 to 1942 I paid the Council the sum of one **dollar** per month for the building that I used as a clinic for treating cancer patients. I treated thousands of patients who came from far and near, most of them given up as hopeless after everything in medical science had failed. Some arrived in ambulances and being too weak to walk into the clinic, they received their first treatments in the ambulance. After a few treatments they walked into the clinic without help."

ESSIAC is a herbal formula that has been in use since 1922. The formula was given to nurse Rene Caisse from a Canadian Ojibwa Indian. She used it to help people with serious illnesses. Born in Bracebridge, Ontario, Nurse Caisse prepared her original herbal formula into a drink named Essiac, which is Nurse Caisse's name spelled backwards. She said that it cured cancer. From 1922 to 1978, Nurse Caisse helped thousands of people with her Essiac herbal supplement at her clinic in Bracebridge, Ontario, Canada. Although she refused payments for her services, she accepted donations to help support her clinic. The herbs that compose the Tea are Burdock Root, Slippery Elm, Sheep Sorrel and Turkey Rhubarb Root.

On a fateful day in 1922 Canadian nurse Rene Caisse noticed scar tissue on the breast of an elderly English woman. The woman said that doctors had diagnosed her with breast cancer years before. However, the woman didn't want to risk surgery nor did she have the money for it. She had met an old Indian medicine man in the 1890s who told her that he could cure her cancer with an herbal tea. The woman took the medicine man's advice, and consequently she was still alive thirty years later and passed on this herbal remedy to Nurse Caisse.

About a year later, Rene Caisse was walking beside a retired doctor who pointed to a common weed and stated: "Nurse Caisse, if people would use this weed there would be little cancer in the world. Rene later stated: "He told me the name of the plant. It was one of the herbs my patient named as an ingredient of the Indian medicine man's tea. The "weed" was *sheep sorrel*. In a 1974 letter to Dr. Chester Stock of the Memorial Sloan-Kettering Cancer Institute, Rene Caisse stated: "Who in the world would ever think to find a solution to cancer in a common meadow?"

In 1924 she decided to test the tea on her aunt who had cancer of the stomach and was given about six months to live. Her aunt lived for another twenty-one years, cancer free.

Rene Caisse later gave the tea to her 72 year old mother who was diagnosed with inoperable cancer of the liver, with only days to live. Her mother recovered and lived without cancer for another 18 years.

In the ensuing years Nurse Caisse refined and perfected the original "medicine man's" formula. She tested various herbal combinations on laboratory mice and on human cancer patients. She eventually reduced the tea to four herbs: burdock root, sheep sorrel (whole herb including the roots), slippery elm and turkey rhubarb. She called the formula Essiac, which is her surname spelled backwards.

Rene Caisse devoted over fifty years of her life to treating hundreds of cancer patients with Essiac. So effective were her treatments that in 1938 her supporters gathered 55,000 signatures to petition the government to allow Rene Caisse to continue treating cancer patients. A bill was introduced in the Ontario legislature to (allegedly) "authorize Rene Caisse to practice medicine in the Province of Ontario in the treatment of cancer and conditions therein".

Due to the "questionable" machinations of the medical establishment, the bill failed to pass by three votes.

When You Walk Through A Storm

Hold Your Head Up High

And Don't Be Afraid Of The Dark

At The End Of The Storm

There's A Golden Sky

And A Sweet Silver Song Of The Lark

Walk On Through The Wind

Walk On Through The Rain

Though Your Dreams Be Tossed And Blown

Walk On, Walk On With Hope In Your Heart

And You'll Never Walk Alone

You'll Never Walk Alone

These poignant lyrics were written and composed by Rogers and Hammerstein 1945

John Gabriel

Chapter Five

The Slow Murdering of Humanity

It was during my search for uncontaminated foods that I was made realize the utter madness of farming practices in North America. However, people are fighting back. A good number of farmers are moving back to natural growing and harvesting. It is encouraging but, unfortunately, a good way behind the European way of doing things. The Europeans had the insight and gumption to prevent the like of Monsanto to plant their filthy seeds in their countries. Even though a number of those governments were paid off by Monsanto the voice of the people was heard loud and clear. Nineteen European countries have opted out of being part of Monsanto's poisonous agenda. It is part of the New World Order's way of doing things for the "good of humanity". I can just see it coming. Monsanto, too, is as rotten and corrupt as the Pharmaceutical Cartels, and, in time, they must be brought to heel and made pay for their crimes against humanity. The killing of human beings is simply packaged differently, undetectable for a period of time, maybe years, but when the poisons build and clog the human system the torturous cancerous demise of the body begins. It might well be termed as a "slow genocidal process."

Please, if you are ill with cancer or any other disease stay away from all foods that are pestizied, chemicalized, and poisonized including all processed "stuff". That means most of what you see on the shelves in "food" stores. When you begin to replace poisoned food with clean, natural food you will feel much better and in a short while you will also

come to understand and feel the benefits of vegetables grown in God's natural earth, especially those grown locally.

REMEMBER HOMICIDE: IT EQUATES WITH PESTICIDES, FUNGICIDES, INSECTICIDES, INFANTICIDE, AND ALL OTHER "CIDES" ASSOCIATED WITH THE DESTRUCTION AND MURDER OF THE FARM SOIL AND THE PEOPLE WHO CONSUME SUCH POISONOUS FOODS.

Health food and juicing became an important part of my therapy. I was drawn to the Champion Juicer because it is built to last and do a good job. However, for me, they were too expensive—four hundred dollars for a fellow on a small pension was a bit much, but also recommended was part two of the juicer—the press. The press was designed to squeeze the heck out of the pulp to obtain forty percent more juice. With both parts of the juicer I was looking at fourteen hundred dollars with the exchange rate, taxes, and postal service. The Canadian dollar was at and still is at one of its common miserable lows. However, not to discourage the buyer or seeker, there are many juicers on the market that do a great job. I went on Kijji, and lo and behold, I spotted a Champion Juicer for the good price of one-seventy-five Canadian dollars. It was a good buy, but for sure it had been used a lot more that I had hoped. However, after a bit of experimenting with the juicer I got the hang of things. A press was not needed because I ran the pulp through a number of times (five or six times) and extracted maximum juice. Nevertheless, there are a great many juicers of different names brands and types that will do the job and they are competitively priced—a little over a hundred dollars to just under two hundred dollars will yield a good juicer. Also, one can check out Kijji. For sure, a juicer can be obtained for next to nothing that will do the job. There are essentially two types of juicers: centrifugal and masticating. The Champion is a masticator, but either one will do. As my search for things to cure my cancer intensified I took notice of the many products that claimed effectiveness in preventing cancer. Having the disease made me susceptible to purchase just about anything that made such a claim and pretty soon my shelf was filled with products of great promises. Unfortunately, I am not a wise shopper, and with the fear of cancer and dying running through my head incessantly made me the perfect fool to purchase any product that made such claims—and there are many. Please be careful—vigilant. But one can hardly go wrong with juicing.

Nothing tastes more delicious than freshly squeezed vegetables and fruit. Maximum benefits are utilized from the juicing. I eventually got around to experimenting with an array of fruits and vegetables and also found it enjoyable to shop for nutritious foods. It was a good study as well as good exercise. There were fruits and vegetables that I had never heard of because I was programmed to eating the foods of my childhood: potatoes, cabbage, lettuce, carrots and beets; onions, celery and sprouts and an array of herbs. They were grown in our garden which supplied us with fresh organic veggies most of the year.

The insane invasion into God's realm with genetically altered farm produce and the chemicalized destruction of the pure land by armies of insane, corrupted so-called scientists were yet to be formed. Although born into abject poverty and a family of twelve, my parents knew the value of fresh veggies and fruits. Even in winter, from other lands, came fresh foods, foods that were not Monsantoized (genetically altered). Although times were tough for my parents, they saw to it that good foods were supplied to their hungry charges. We ate healthy and kept healthy—most of the time, but there was always that craving for "sweet things".

John Gabriel

There Are No Excuses

Chapter Six

Deadly Sugar

Sugar, in most cases, is added to the morning cup of coffee or tea. It is baked into pastries, cakes, and cookies, and even sprinkled over breakfast cereal for added "flavor." It's hidden in some beloved "treats" that people consume on a daily basis, such as sodas, fruit juices, candies, and ice cream. It also lurks in almost all processed foods, including breads, meats, and even condiments like Ketchup and a myriad of other sauces and foods. Most people view sugary foods as tasty, satisfying, and irresistible treats. But I believe that there are two words that describe sugar more accurately: **addicting and deadly.**

Sugar is proven to be one of the most damaging substances that one can ingest and what is terrifying about it is its abundance. This intense addiction to sugar is becoming rampant, not just among adults, but in children as well. But how exactly does sugar work in our body, and what are the side effects of eating too much sugar? It is easy to imagine how the consumption of too much sugar can and does settle in on a person as "dead weight". Excess sugar becomes metabolized into body fat leading to all the debilitating diseases many people struggle with. It overloads and damages the liver; it tricks the body into gaining weight and affects one's insulin. In short, like cancer, if not checked in time it eventually kills us. One study found that fructose is readily used by cancer cells to increase their proliferation—it "feeds" the cancer cells, promoting cell division and speeding their growth, which allow the cancer to spread faster. For sure—sugar is not a friend. As is said, everything to moderation, but with sugar the less consumed the better.

Marijuana's Comeback: Today, even though stigma and prejudice exist in regards to the use of marijuana the general mindset is far more relaxed because of some honest medical and political research, and also the uncovering of the great "cover-up" by the pharmaceutical cartels by the like of Carnegie and the Rockefellers. They were instrumental in closing any natural proven cures to cancer, such as Essiac Tea and marijuana, because great profit was to be made in the production of "chemical cures". Chemicals they could patent but not anything derived from nature. Therefore "nature" was their enemy because anything from nature cannot be patented. Today, fifty billion dollars a year profit is made by the Pharmaceutical cartels in the chemical treatment of cancer.

However, fair minded people and nature are fighting back. By twenty-twenty, by the way things are moving, marijuana looks like it will be just another accepted product available at the pharmacy or from the farm grower. There are many claims to the positive results cannabis oil possesses in dealing with a myriad of ailments, but it is in its ability to target and kill cancer cells that is getting a lot of attention worldwide. Because of the positive feed-back, the relief, and claimed cures of this plant, open-minded governments and private agencies globally are becoming more involved in the ongoing study of marijuana for medicinal benefits.

Marijuana, a word and entity steeped in controversy has over the years given an excellent account of its healing abilities. It is slowly making in-roads throughout the medical systems. Some governments and medical agencies are working hand in hand in stripping away the unwise and unfair stigma attached to it. Medical marijuana, up to this point, on human subjects, has not been officially tested for its healing abilities, but from what I am experiencing and witnessing that platform is not too far away. And although in its infant stages in Canada, the medical marijuana enterprise is now morphing into a true realm of healing and it is just a matter of time before all barriers worldwide are sidelined.

As the debate over legalizing marijuana heats up, many continue to dispute the value of marijuana as a treatment for various ailments. But, as the following facts show, history tells a much clearer story.

In 2737 B.C., Chinese Emperor Shennong wrote a book on medicine that included cannabis as a treatment for many conditions. According to ancient Chinese texts, cannabis was thought to be helpful for constipation, rheumatism and absent-mindedness. Interestingly, Shennong was not only an emperor but a pharmacologist as well. He was said to have experimented with hundreds of herbs on himself in order to test their medical value. It is also reported that the ancient Egyptians were the first to use cannabis oil in the treatment of tumors.

The second century Fayyum Medical Papyrus, an ancient Egyptian text, is believed to contain the earliest record of cannabis as an ingredient in cancer medicine.

While little is known about the successes of ancient Egyptian cancer treatments, cannabis continues to receive significant interest as a cancer therapy and cure today. However, the use of cannabis for medical purposes seemed to be well in use in the ancient world. The Greeks, too, used cannabis to dress wounds and sores on their horses after battle. The plant was also given to humans for a variety of ailments, including ear pain and inflammation. In the 1830s, an Irish physician William Brooke O' Shaughnessy observed the use of marijuana during a trip to India. After studying its effects, he introduced cannabis to physicians in England as a treatment for a wide range of conditions, including muscle spasms, rheumatism, epilepsy and pain. As early reports of its effectiveness were published, the popularity of cannabis-based medicines quickly spread across Europe and North America.

By the late 18th century, early editions of American medical journals recommended cannabis seeds and roots for the treatment of inflamed skin, incontinence and venereal disease. Dr. William O'Shaughnessy first popularized marijuana's medical use in Ireland, England and America. As a physician with the British East India Company, he found marijuana eased the pain of rheumatism and was helpful against discomfort and nausea in cases of rabies, cholera and tetanus.

It is important that cannabis oil, also known as "hemp oil" is not confused with hemp-seed-oil. While hemp-<u>seed</u>-oil is used to promote good health it does not cure cancer. Cannabis oil = hemp oil = marijuana oil. Hemp-<u>seed</u>-oil stands alone and is legally available in Canada but in the present is not in the USA.

The following is a procedure in the ingesting of cannabis oil recommended by Rick Simpson, a Canadian who cured his melanoma cancer, a deadly skin disease, with cannabis oil. In fact, he is one of the first people who stood against the so called "authorities" and openly promoted and supported the use of medicinal cannabis for those who were let down by government and the medical establishment.

"People should start by orally ingesting their dose of cannabis oil three times per day. For the first week each total dose should be the size of a half grain of white rice. After the oil has been taken for a week, start to double the dose. The dose should be doubled every four days until 1 gram/ml per day is ingested. Usually, it takes thirty to thirty-five days to prepare the body for the intake of 1 gram/ml per day. Once ingesting one gram/ml of oil per day is achieved, dosage should continue at that rate until the cancer is gone. However, some people have increased their daily doses to two grams or more. Since the initial intake of oil is a relatively small amount, it is convenient for cannabis oil to be fed out of an oral syringe into empty capsules that can be purchased at most health-food stores. This allows for the amount of oil to be consistent and precise for persons of all ages, including children being introduced to the use of cannabis oil **treatment. Oral syringes also make it very easy to store your cannabis oil discreetly.**

According to the Rick Simpson (*online-Rick Simpson Phoenix Tears—Phoneix Tears is just a name for cannabis oil*) method of cancer treatment and cure, sixty ounces of the oil is required to kill off the cancer permanently.

Again, it is important that hemp-<u>seed</u>-oil is not confused with hemp oil (cannabis oil). While hemp-seed-oil is used for promoting beneficial health, it does not cure cancer.

I Will Not Feel Deprived

When I Turn Down Junk Food

I Will Feel Empowered

That I Made A Healthy Choice

From The Web:

General Public Information

And Professional

Medical Advice

On Good Health Practices

Colon cleansing has been used throughout history to detoxify the body and improve the general quality life. In fact, the use of water to cleanse colon has been practiced in ancient Egypt.

The ultimate goal of a colon cleanse is to help the digestive organs do their job in the best way possible, managing things that get in the way and interfere with normal bowel functions. Colon cleanses aren't necessarily needed by every person, but some people can really benefit from eliminating waste, bacterial matter and toxic material that's stored in their bodies.

The colon is home to billions of microflora (bacteria) that actually make up approximately seventy percent of the dry weight of feces. Besides forming stool, the various beneficial bacterial organisms living within the colon and digestive tract are important for proper nutrient absorption, maintaining proper pH balance, controlling hunger and counteracting potentially dangerous bacteria. This is the reason that a well-functioning colon is essential for overall well-being.

While the digestive system has its own processes for removing waste, many people struggle with having regular, complete bowel movements due to various reasons like poor gut health, allergies, consumption of pesticide chemicals and inflammation within the digestive system.

Irritable bowel movement is estimated to affect about 15 percent to 20 percent of the adult population worldwide, while chronic constipation is one of the most common gastrointestinal problems in the world, affecting about forty-two million people in the U.S. alone. These problems are especially common among people with poor diets, women during pregnancy, older adults, people recovering from surgery and those taking medications.

One needs to have at least one bowel movement every day, this makes for a good colon cleanse. It's well-known that a variety of health problems stem from poor digestive health. For example, stomach pains, abdominal cramps, chronic fatigue, constipation, low energy, headaches and allergic reactions can all be traced back partially to problems with waste elimination.

An impacted bowel can easily cause sluggishness, irritation, irritability and low energy. That's because unreleased food and waste particles can cause mucus and bacteria to ferment and form in the colon, which might result in toxins being released back into the bloodstream. Failing to have regular bowel movements also poses the risk for problems absorbing nutrients properly, which can lead to low energy and other complications.

The colon is the longest part of the large intestine, which is attached to the small intestine at one end and the anus at the other. The task of the colon is to eliminate stool from the body that is made up of a combination of bacteria, water, unused nutrients, unneeded electrolytes and digested food. There are many different methods for performing a colon cleanse, which sometimes go under the names colonic, colonic irrigation, colon therapy or colonic hydrotherapy. You can also effectively flush the colon doing a juice fast, salt water flush, or performing an enema. Colon cleanses are split into two main categories: one type requires that a professional perform the cleanse, while the other involves using a solution or supplement at home.

One of the most common reasons someone would have a colonic done by a professional is because he or she is preparing for surgery or a medical procedure (such as colonoscopy) that requires the colon to be completely clear from accumulated waste. On the other hand, cleansing is commonly done at home using an enema, laxatives or herbal supplements.

Many colon cleanses work by inserting a tube into the rectum followed by large amounts of water, which makes its way through the colon. The water carries out any matter that might be dry and lodged in place. The exact amount of water or other type of liquid that's used depends on the specific type of colon-cleansing method. Colonics, for example, can use up to sixteen gallons (about sixty liters) of water at one time.

While there's plenty of anecdotal evidence, considering colon cleanses have been done since Ancient Egyptian times. Millions of people over the years have found relief from doing colon cleanses, and when done safely and correctly, they shouldn't pose any risks. For people who haven't found lasting relief from things like laxatives or prescriptions, a colon cleanse can finally help bring about regular bowel movements and decrease symptoms.

Studies show that bowel movements are important for removing bacteria and eliminating excess fatty acids from the body. A colon cleanse can also impact the nervous system positively, which is why it might help symptoms like anxiety and fatigue.

A clogged colon can affect one's mood. That's because nerves in the bowel communicate to the brain and affect chemical signals sent via the entire central nervous system throughout the body. A well-functioning colon therefore is important for hormonal balance, appetite control, sleep and mental processing.

Certain enemas might also be able to help the body absorb nutrients better. When doing a colon cleanse using coffee, for example, antioxidants and caffeine travel via the hemorrhoidal vein to the liver. Together, they can help open up blood vessels, improve circulation, relax smooth muscles that control bowel movements, and increase production of bile that's needed for proper digestion and excretion.

Colon cleanses and colonics can take anywhere from 20–90 minutes, depending on which kind you decide to try. Some people react more quickly and experience better results than others, but keep in mind that colon cleanses might become more effective and easier the more often you do them. At first, it might seem difficult to insert much liquid and hold it in, but you might find colon cleanses become more beneficial as you learn how to do them properly with practice.

To understand the different options you have in regard to various colon cleanses, it helps to have some background of how different types work and affect the digestive system. Keep in mind that water isn't the only substance used during colon cleansing. Various saline formulas, herbs or acidic solutions are also used to flush waste.

Here are the basics of how popular colon cleanse techniques work: Colonics have been performed for over one hundred years and are done by hygienists or colon hydrotherapists. These treatments are sometimes called "colon irrigation" and are normally done at a treatment center outside the home.

Colonics use a high quantity of water to flush the colon. They usually require the most water of all colon cleanses — for example, about the same amount you'd use if you performed 12 enemas.

Of all colon cleanses, they're thought to be one of the most productive and thorough, since they target the entire colon. The drawback is that they're performed by a professional outside the home and take about one to two hours in total for each session. This can become costly since each session can cost fifty dollars or more.

There are several types of colonics available, including those that use gravity and pressurized machines. A gravity colonic is the most basic and uses water that enters the colon by force of gravity, as opposed to a machine. Gravity colonics are done by controlling the in and out flow of water into the rectum while massaging the abdomen to help break up stool and encourage the muscles to relax and release.

During a colonic you lay flat on a table and the professional inserts a lubricated, small speculum (a metal or plastic instrument that is used to dilate an orifice or canal in the body to allow inspection) into your colon, which is attached to two tubes that control the release of water in and out. Often you will be left alone, given the option to help control the release of the liquid yourself. You might also be able to view what's coming out if you'd like to. After the colonic is over, you can use the bathroom until you're comfortable. Pressurized colonics are different than gravity-controlled ones because the flow is controlled by a machine, which makes them a bit less gentle.

Colonic procedures are quiet different from that of an enema. Compared to colonics, which are done at a clinic and the under supervision of a professional, enemas can be performed at home in private. This makes enemas an attractive option for people who aren't very comfortable with the idea of visiting a specialist for this matter. They're also inexpensive, and kits can be bought at any drug store.

Enemas work by cleansing the colon with liquid (usually water), which helps flush out accumulated waste. Compared to colonics, they're usually milder and target a specific region of the colon (the left side, or descending colon) as opposed to the whole colon. It's easiest and most common to perform an enema with water, but you can also do one using a saline solution such as apple cider vinegar, hydrogen peroxide or even green coffee (not everyday use coffee. For a full understanding of coffee enemas look up the Gerson Cancer Center: **Gerson Therapy Non-Toxic Cancer Immunotherapy_issels.com**

To perform an enema, you insert the pointed tip into your own colon, control the release of liquid, and then lay down and wait until you have the urge to use the bathroom, which might happen several times over the course of one to two hours. Along with enemas, hydrotherapy works wonders for the body, mind and spirit.

Hydrotherapy is the term for "the use of water to treat a disease or to maintain health." The idea behind hydrotherapy is that water itself has healing abilities, and when combined with other substances like coffee or salt, it also supplies essential nutrients like various antioxidants or trace minerals. The use of water in hydrotherapy to cleanse the colon is basically the same as an enema or colonic. The water helps expel waste, can relieve constipation, improve energy levels, treat dehydration and sometimes provide important minerals safely.

Baking soda is really an astonishing friend to mankind. Cancer cells have a lower pH than surrounding tissues. Sodium bicarbonate cancer treatments work by increasing pH. As if it were not humiliating enough for orthodox oncologists to learn that the lowly chemical sodium bicarbonate (baking soda) is important in the treatment of cancer now they have to swallow the research pointing to the fact that bicarbonate can also be used to diagnose cancer in its earliest stages. Oncologists do understand and know that bicarbonate is necessary to protect their patients from the toxicity and harm done by highly toxic chemicals used in chemotherapy. They also know it is of extraordinary help to patients receiving radiation treatments protecting as it does the kidneys and other tissues of the body from radioactive damage.

Oncologists should also know that bicarbonate induced extracellular alkalinization leads to significant improvements in the therapeutic effectiveness of certain chemo agents. A number of studies have shown that the extracellular pH in cancers is typically lower than that in normal tissue and that an **acidic pH promotes invasive tumor growth in primary and metastatic cancers.** The external pH of solid tumors is acidic as a consequence of increased metabolism of glucose and poor perfusion.

Researchers have investigated the very reasonable assumption that increased systemic concentrations of pH buffers would lead to reduced intratumoral and peritumoral acidosis and, as a result, inhibit malignant growth. It has been shown that increased serum concentrations of the sodium bicarbonate can be achieved via oral intake. These researchers found that consequent reduction of tumor acid concentrations significantly reduces tumor growth and invasion without altering the pH of blood or normal tissues. It is known that bicarbonate turns to CO2 easily when dissolved in water as it enters the stomach but few know that **cancerous tissue turns bicarbonate into carbon dioxide**. A few years ago a United Kingdom Cancer Research team found MRI scans were able to track changes in bicarbonate and therefore identify cancers even in the very early stages.

All cancer has a lower pH, meaning it is more acidic than surrounding tissue. Working with mice, the researchers boosted the MRI sensitivity more than twenty thousand times. Using MRI, they looked to see how much of the tagged bicarbonate was converted into carbon dioxide within the tumor. In more acidic tumors, more bicarbonate is converted into carbon dioxide.

Lead researcher Professor Kevin Brindle, from Cancer Research UK's Cambridge Research Institute at the University of Cambridge, said: "This technique could be used as a highly-sensitive early warning system for the signs of cancer. By exploiting the body's natural pH balancing system, we have found a potentially safe way of measuring pH to see what's going on inside patients. MRI can pick up on the abnormal pH levels found in cancer and it is possible that this could be used to pinpoint where the disease is present and when it is responding to treatment."

Given its alkalizing (or basic) pH of approximately 9.0, baking soda counteracts the acidity that accumulates in the body. Baking soda is useful to regulate by buffering the pH of cells, tissues, and voltage homeostasis within cells. It is also useful to increase oxygenation and carbon dioxide. **Baking soda can also be used to aid the body in the detoxification process** and support the body in healing from radiation exposure and oxidative damage.

Natural health care practitioners utilize sodium bicarbonate to defend against numerous health ailments. Some of these include the common cold, kidney diseases, diabetes, the flu, and some even use baking soda to treat cancer. When used as a bath soak, the body can absorb the health benefits of baking soda through the skin. It can also be used as a nebulizer to treat lung conditions.

Each tumor is distinguished by its own unique traits and all may not be extremely acidic. Regardless of the tumors acidity, balancing and creating a slightly alkaline internal body environment is beneficial to the patient's internal systems. Ideally, pH strip testing should result between 7.0 and 8.0. **If a reading higher than 8.0 results, discontinue baking soda use immediately until pH decreases**.

Testing and monitoring both urine and saliva pH should be used in conjunction with sodium bicarbonate treatments. You can do this with a pH test or an electronic tester. Test every morning and chart the results. Test both urinary and salivary pH when you get out of a bath with baking soda. Again, if the pH climbs above 8.0, stop use of baking soda treatments until the pH lowers.

Unmonitored use of baking soda therapy can have health hazards. Some of these consequences include reduced stomach pH concentration, kidney complications, alkalosis, etc. To avoid these dangers be responsible with use and take the time to chart your pH levels throughout your day. Avoid consuming baking soda within 30 minutes of a meal to limit digestive problems.

The Baking Soda Drink: Only consume this drink when you have tested your pH throughout the day and your results are acidic. As a reminder, do not drink this beverage 30 minutes before or after a meal to avoid lowering stomach acid secretions and inhibiting proper digestion. This beverage will aid in neutralizing pH, buffer stomach acid, and lower acidosis. Drink the following mixture throughout the day except before and after meals until your pH levels are stabilized between 7.0 and 8.0.

Ingredients:

Tall glass

½ tsp baking soda

2 tbs fresh lemon juice

8 oz. purified water

Directions: Mix baking soda with fresh lemon juice or organic apple cider vinegar. The combination will result in a foam or fizz. This is normal.

Once all bubbling has stopped, add water to the mixture and drink all at once.

This information is being suppressed from you by the mainstream media and the medical establishment. Please share this information with friends and family. It could save someone's life!

A cancer research team in the U.K. is developing a technique that uses baking soda in conjunction with a highly sensitive MRI scan to identify cancer cell growth. It appears that presently significant advances are been made in discovering very promising treatments of cancer and all seem to associate with nature's way: cannabis oil, Essiac Tea, baking Soda—vitamin B17. Cannabis Oil cured my cancer but today I include all of the above to ward off any possibility of a comeback.

If you decide to include baking soda in your healing protocol, make sure to purchase Bob's Red Mill baking Soda as it is all natural or any brand of baking soda available in a health food store. Commercial brands are processed using aluminum, the last thing you want in your system. And one last word of good advice: use only steel kitchenware to do the cooking. Aluminum pots and pans are a danger to one's health as with each use of the utensil aluminum taints the food and over time builds in the body. For cheap stuff, we pay sooner or later and, at times, the cost is extremely high.

Thank you for taking time to read about my experience with cancer. It is my sincere wish that you might find some information that will assist you or a loved one in the battle against cancer and other illnesses. Some statements—excerpts—have been borrowed from the internet under the **"fair use"** agreement to give a clear, concise understanding of natures' remedies in curing cancer and other serious ailments. The list is as follows and is well worth taking note and making study: The following links present a story of Canada's most noble and brilliant nurse, Rene Caisse and her battle against corrupt noodles in governments and the pharmaceutical cartels. Nevertheless, she cured thousands of terminally ill patients and gave to the world a well proven cure for all cancers.

Cancer cure:http:/www.youtube.com/watch/v=wch9d yLEccg

The story of Essiac Tea: http://www.youtube.com/watch?v=jojYLUwS jhI

Five reasons why Essiac tea should be used for optimum health: It is an excellent presentation on the natural properties of the tea and how it works

https://www.youtube.com/watch?v=9ory2-oJIeo

This man is amazing. He had exactly the same cancer that I had. Whereas he had the operation and refused chemo and radiation, I had chemo and radiation but not the operation. We both lived to tell our stories. Please take time to listen to this wonderful, dedicated man and his amazing story.

Chrisbeatcancer.https://www.youtube.com/watch?v=_k3B0y0tjCg

Amazing: Hemp oil (cannabis oil) cured this man's stage 4 pancreatic cancer. There are literally hundred of testimonials given to the remarkable power of cannabis oil in curing cancer—and I am one of those people.

https://www.youtube.com/watch?v=vZN1-_lBaxo

Baking soda and molasses cure for cancer:

https://www.youtube.com/watch?v=ENk84KHUs1M

The power of apple seeds in killing cancer:

https://www.youtube.com/watch?v=GrJEqNdkCjw

Healing cancer with apricot seeds and the truth about pharmaceutical companies.

https://www.youtube.com/watch?v=dNjMdbUb5gU&t=67s

Above are links to natural cancer treatments and cures shown on youtube by medical professionals and victims of this scourge. Just for convenience, the links are my choice, but there are many "eye-opening" presentations that one can study and research. We do have choices; let's use them wisely. Cure your cancer and live happily and free of pain.

"In the world of plants there is a cure for every ailment and disease known to man." Edgar Cayce, The Sleeping Prophet.

Edgar Cayce was almost a hundred years ahead of his time in holistic medicine. In fact, many people presently in that field use his remedies in all kinds of treatments. His videos and writings can be seen freely on Youtube. His story, more incredible than that of Nostradamus is well worth watching.

In the early nineteen-hundreds cancer struck one person in twenty. In 1970 it was one person in sixteen. Today, it strikes one person in three and the latest news from the Canadian Cancer

Society is that one in two will suffer the curse of cancer in the very near future.

The chemicalized foods that we ingest indeed do kill us.

John Gabriel

WORK THIS OUT

ALCOHOL

Addictive, Depressant;

Causes Millions of Deaths Each Year

Costs Police and NHS Billions

Death via O.D.

Endless Crimes Due to Its Abuse--LEGAL

CANNABIS

Non Addictive; Anti Depressant

Cures Cancer; Zero Deaths in History

Saves Police and NHS Billions

No O.D.

Grows Brain Cells—ILLEGAL

The Gerson Therapy

Also World Renowned For its

Success in Treating

And Curing Cancer

"I see in him one of the most eminent geniuses in the history of medicine. Many of his basic ideas have been adopted without having his name connected with them. Yet, he has achieved more than seemed possible under adverse conditions. He leaves a legacy which commands attention and which will assure him his due place. Those whom he has cured will now attest to the truth of his ideas."

~ Albert Schweitzer, MD (Nobel Peace Prize Winner, 1952)

Who was Albert Schweitzer talking about? He was referring to Dr. Max Gerson, the German-born American medical doctor who developed one of the most effective natural cancer treatments over 90 years ago. Coined the "**Gerson Therapy**," Dr. Gerson helped hundreds of cancer patients activate their body's extraordinary ability to heal itself by recommending:

- Organic, plant-based foods
- Raw juices
- **Coffee enemas**
- Beef liver
- Natural supplements

In the words of the Gerson Institute:

With its whole-body approach to healing, the Gerson Therapy naturally reactivates your body's magnificent ability to heal itself — with no damaging side effects. This a powerful, natural treatment boosts the body's own immune system to heal cancer, arthritis, heart disease, allergies, and many other degenerative diseases.

The Gerson Therapy targets the most significant metabolic requirements in your body. How? Believe it or not, this therapy allows you to reap the nutritional benefits of consuming 15–20 pounds of organically grown fruits and vegetables each day! Here's the breakdown:

The Gerson Diet:– Consisting of eating only organic fruits, vegetables and sprouted ancient grains, the Gerson Diet is exceptionally rich in vitamins, minerals and enzymes. It's also very low in fats, proteins and sodium. The meal plan advises cancer patients to drink 13 glasses of freshly prepared juice, eat three plant-based meals, and only snack on fresh fruits each day. Also, the traditional Gerson Therapy recommends consuming raw beef liver since it is the most nutrient-dense food on the planet and extremely high in vitamin B12.

Juicing: According to the Gerson Institute, "Fresh pressed juice from raw foods provides the easiest and most effective way of providing high quality nutrition." The cancer-fighting protocol calls for patients to drink fresh vegetables each day, including raw carrots or apples and green-leaf juice. To preserve the nutritional content, the juice should be prepared hourly using a two-step juicer or a masticating juicer used with a separate hydraulic press. This helps prevent denaturation—when vitamins, minerals and enzymes are destroyed. (Most commercial juicers spin so fast that they heat up juice to the point they are basically pasteurized!)

Detoxification– The Gerson Therapy utilizes coffee enemas as the primary method of detoxing the body by increasing the parasympathetic nervous system. For cancer patients, this may take up to five enemas each day. The importance of keeping the body free of toxins is paramount and coffee enemas can play a superb role in doing just that.

You might consider yourself a true "coffee lover" who knows all the **coffee nutrition facts**, but would you be willing to try an unconventional way of using coffee to improve your health? While *drinking* coffee has its well-documented benefits, that's not the only way to reap the rewards of this antioxidant-packed beverage. While it might sound strange to inject the caffeinated liquid directly into your colon, research shows that coffee enemas are an effective way to clean out the lower intestines and improve your health.

Coffee enemas are known to help flush out bacteria, heavy metals, fungus and yeast (like those responsible for candida symptoms, for example) from the digestive tract, including the liver and colon, while also lowering inflammation—therefore helping people restore bowel function, increase their energy levels and heal from disorders that have caused them trouble for years.

Before you start thinking that this sounds completely crazy, consider the fact that various types of natural detoxification treatments, including enemas, have been used for thousands of years to help restore digestive function and general health. Some were even mentioned in ancient historical scripts like The Dead Sea Scrolls that described how Jesus used ordinary ingredients and materials, like food and water, to help heal illnesses.

Various types of natural enemas, even **fecal transplants** or other ways of unconventionally restoring gut health, are growing in popularity as more people realize that laxatives and prescriptions fail to address the underlying cause of digestive disorders.

While still not exactly a mainstream way to fight illness, coffee enemas are nothing new. They've been around since the late 1800s and were used at the time to help speed up healing following surgeries or to combat cases of accidental poisoning. First made famous by the Gerson Institute in the 1950s, when it began using coffee enemas as a key to treating cancer patients, others are now turning to this procedure for various ailments that don't respond well to traditional treatments or prescription medications.

Today, doctors of functional and alternative medicines use coffee enemas as part of natural treatment protocols for fighting cancer, parasites, overdoses, constipation, liver dysfunction, candida virus, IBS and other digestive disorders.

How do coffee enemas work? According to the Gerson Institute, they have the primary purpose of "removing toxins accumulated in the liver and removing free radicals from the bloodstream." And it's not just the caffeine in coffee that is responsible for the benefits of coffee enemas; in fact, studies show that bioavailability of caffeine obtained from coffee enemas is about 3.5 times less than those obtained drinking coffee orally.

It's well known that coffee beans naturally contain antioxidants and beneficial compounds, including cafestol-palmitate, kahweol, theobromine, theophylline in addition to caffeine, that have positive effects on inflammation levels, including within the digestive system. When ingested, compounds within coffee either from drinking it or from inserting coffee directly into the colon act like a cathartic that causes the colon muscles to contract. This helps move along stool through the digestive tract, resolving cases of constipation and making it easier to go to the bathroom.

As you're probably aware, regular bowel movements are beneficial for carrying waste and toxins (like heavy metals or excess fatty acids) out of the body. Research has shown, then, during a coffee enema caffeine and other compounds travel via the hemorrhoidal vein to the liver. Coffee opens up blood vessels, relaxes smooth muscles that help with bowel movements and improves circulation. Once it makes its way to the liver, coffee is also believed to help open up bile ducts and increase production of bile that's needed for proper digestion and excretion.

Researchers from the University of Minnesota also demonstrated that coffee enema benefits might include being able to help stimulate the production of a beneficial enzyme created in the liver called **glutathione** S-transferase, which acts like a antioxidant, anti-inflammatory and natural blood cleanser. (6) Some evidence shows that coffee enemas can help with:

- repairing digestive tissue
- cleansing the liver
- improving blood circulation
- increasing immunity
- helping with cellular regeneration

- relieving digestive issues, such as frequent constipation, bloating, cramping and nausea
- improving gut health
- improving low energy levels and moods (such as fighting signs of depression)

Coffee enemas are believed to increase production of glutathione S-transferase above normal levels. As functional medicine practitioner and pharmacist Suzy Cohen points out, people pay good money for glutathione in supplement form, so having the ability to produce more on your own is pretty valuable!

What makes this enzyme so powerful is its ability to scavenge free radicals within the digestive tract that contribute to bodywide inflammation, poor gut health, **liver disease** and cellular damage. Once free radicals are neutralized, bile that is produced from the liver and gallbladder carries these substances out of the body through bowel movements.

Max Gerson, M.D., author of "A Cancer Therapy," which was published in 1958, has successfully used coffee enemas in thousands of cancer patients. (8) Dr. Gerson made coffee enemas famous as a **natural cancer treatment** when he pioneered the use of a special anti-inflammatory diet combined with nutritional supplements and daily enemas for speeding up detoxification.

According to the National Cancer Institute, an organic vegetarian diet plus pancreatic enzymes and coffee enemas were the main features of the Gerson Therapy that intended to build up the immune system of cancer patients and restore electrolyte balance (such as levels of potassium in cells). Many of his patients were able to stop their pain medications and help restore liver function and tissue repair by performing sometimes up to six coffee enemas per day.

Acting similarly to "a form of dialysis of the blood," coffee enemas help remove unwanted materials from the gut wall and bloodstream. Dialysis is considered a forced or artificial method to enhance detoxification, and that's exactly what coffee edemas do since they help the body expel waste materials. The primarily role of the enema is to mechanically wash out the colon, removing potentially harmful parasites, bacteria, yeast and heavy metals that contribute to inflammation and therefore disease.

There's some evidence that coffee acts like a natural "astringent," since it helps the top layer of skin or mucous membranes within the digestive tract peel off and rejuvenate (similarly to how astringents used on skin help with cell turnover). Some researchers believe that the top layer of mucous within the gut lining might hold a high level of toxins, and therefore, helping the body shed this lining speeds up the cleansing process.

Aside from the coffee itself, there's also therapeutic effects of the water used in coffee enemas. Water therapy, known as hydrotherapy, helps the body heal by flushing the colon and rectum while also speeding up transit time of stool.

Constipation is one of the most common problems for adults, which is why laxatives are one of the most widely purchased over-the-counter medicines there is. If you're one of millions of adults who struggle to **poop** regularly, you'll be happy to know that coffee enemas provide **natural constipation relief** in several ways. First off, the increase in water that is inserted into the colon helps stimulate peristalsis in the gut, while a portion of the water also helps increase bile production.

The mechanical effects of the enema cause the colon to become more active and facilitate the emptying of stool and removing of impacted feces, toxins and food residues that can cause constipation. Coffee might also help clean out diverticuli in the colon, which are slight openings in the colon wall that can cause left-behind food particles or bacterial organisms to become trapped.

People usually experience the best results from coffee enemas when they also drink plenty of water and improve their diets, such as cutting out inflammatory foods like sugar, white refined flour and hydrogenated fats that can slow down digestion.

Coffee enemas can be assembled and performed easily and inexpensively at home in the comfort of your own bathroom (or wherever you choose). To perform a coffee enema at home, you need to purchase an enema kit along with fresh coffee beans. Enema kits can be found in certain health food or drug stores, and definitely online. There are several types available, from simpler versions that are sometimes called "traveler's kits" to plastic bucket types that use gravity to help the enema work better. No matter the type you use, look for one that has a tube and nozzle attached to either a bucket or bag that hangs above you when you lie down.

After choosing a enema kit, you need to purchase coffee beans. You want to purchase only certified organic coffee and regular (not decaf) beans that are free from all chemical sprays—this is important considering the quality of the coffee determines how effective the detoxification process will be. The last thing you want to do is directly insert chemicals into your digestive tract if you already deal with inflammation and dysfunction! Most people recommend keeping your coffee beans in the freezer until you're ready to perform the enema so they retain the most antioxidants.

As with all enemas, it's best to do one immediately after having a bowel movement if possible, which makes it more comfortable, effective and easier to retain for longer. You can also do an enema even if you haven't recently had a bowel movement (for example, if you're constipated), but many people like to perform enemas in the morning directly after going to the bathroom.

It's recommended to do an enema about once weekly or up to once daily if you're healing from a digestive disorder. In fact, in some cases very ill patients (for example, people healing from cancer) have used coffee enemas multiple times per day. If you choose to do coffee enemas frequently, you might want to consider buying a reusable enema kit and cleaning the nozzle with a natural detergent to save money.

Once you have your materials prepared, here is a step-by-step guide to follow in order to perform a coffee enema safely:

1. Proceed with caution.
2. To make one enema, use a small pot on your stove top to combine coffee beans with filtered water. Filtered water is highly recommended by most experts and might offer fewer risks than tap water

(which contain traces of minerals or chemicals). Add 2 tablespoons of organic coffee beans to your pot along with 3 cups of filtered water. Then bring to a boil and let simmer for 15 minutes.

3. Let the mixture cool down to a little warmer than room temperature once it's boiled for about 15 minutes. Strain the coffee beans from the mixture so you have one uniform liquid free from particles.

4. You're now ready to perform your enema, so choose a location that's comfortable where you can lie down for about 15 minutes, such as the bathroom floor with some towels. Most people like to be close to a toilet and keep extra towels on hand to clean up if need be. Wherever you choose to be, take your enema kit and place the bucket or bag at least 1 meter above you and the ground. So if you're lying on the floor, you might try hanging the bucket or bag on a towel rack, shower rail, etc. This helps gravity push the coffee liquid down

faster so it's better able to enter your digestive tract and do its job.

5. Pour your coffee liquid into the enema bag or bucket and hold the tube and nozzle shut. Locate the lever on the tube and nozzle that helps you stop and start the flow of the enema. Before beginning, make sure the valve is shut so no liquid escapes. Use a lubricant such as coconut oil to coat the tip of the enema nozzle, which will make it easier to insert into your rectum without being uncomfortable. Lay down on your right side in fetal position and insert the nozzle into your rectum, aiming for it to be about 1 inch inside.

6. Use the valve that helps you to start the flow of coffee and keep the liquid slowly entering your rectum through the nozzle until the bag or bucket is emptied. Take your time and squeeze in so the liquid doesn't escape as much as possible. Sit however you are most comfortable that helps you keep the coffee inside of you for about 12 to 15 minutes—15 minutes is the max time that

you need to effectively cleanse your system, so at this point you can stop holding in and can go to the bathroom.

Proceed with caution: The Institute of Digestive Disease and Nutrition at the University of Korea has studied the effects of coffee enemas in various patients and reports that people using coffee enemas don't usually experience any complications or side effects. Coffee enemas are considered a safe and feasible option for treating digestive dysfunction, and there were no clinically significant adverse events related to coffee enemas demonstrated at this time.

If you've experienced complications from using enemas in the past, it's best to talk to a doctor before trying to perform a coffee enema on your own. The first time you try a coffee enema it's a good idea to do so under supervision or with guidance of a medical professional, although some people feel comfortable jumping right into the process. Coffee enemas aren't usually recommended for pregnant women or children since they can be sensitive to the effects of caffeine.

Still, all enemas come with certain side effects, including tears in the colon and dehydration or **electrolyte imbalances** if they're over-performed. One way to make the process more comfortable is to always use a lubricant, go very slowly and to follow directions very carefully. Make sure you avoid burns and irritation by cooling the coffee liquid enough and straining it well.

If you've experienced hemorrhoids or tears in the past, you might find inserting the nozzle painful and should not force the procedure. You also don't want to perform more than one enema weekly until you monitor your reactions and make sure you aren't experiencing any signs of dehydration, such as dizziness, muscle cramps or weakness, due to increased bowel movements. Drink plenty of water when using enemas to help flush your system. And please remember what the great philosopher and physician said. **"All Disease Begins In The Gut"-Hippocrates.**

The ancient Greek physician certainly wasn't wrong. In fact, more and more studies are finding that gut issues are the root cause of autoimmune and other diseases, the biggest culprit being leaky gut.

If you experience excessive fatigue, bloating, joint pains, skin problems, and have strong cravings for sugar and carbs, chances are you have a leaky gut, especially when you suddenly become sensitive to certain foods.

Imagine your gut is a house and your gut lining acts as a "gatekeeper," with tight junctions in place to prevent unnecessary or potentially harmful particles from entering your bloodstream. When leaky gut occurs, it's as if the gatekeeper skipped town and left the gate open for anything to pass through.

When the tight junctions in your gut lining break down and become more permeable, random particles can enter your bloodstream. Since these substances aren't meant to leave your digestive tract, your body will set off "alarm bells" to tell your immune system that foreign invaders have entered your bloodstream— much like how a house alarm would call the police if someone broke into your house.

To get these particles out of your body, your immune system reacts aggressively and attacks these particles by eliciting an immune response. While this is intended to protect you, each time an immune response is triggered, it causes inflammation. This is a problem because chronic inflammation is one of the leading causes of many chronic health conditions, such **as heart disease and diabetes.**

In a nutshell, when the tight junctions of your gut (intestinal) lining separate and create "holes" that allow food particles and toxins to pass easily through, that forms a leaky gut.

Those food particles and toxins then pass into your bloodstream which can wreak total havoc on your body causing food intolerances, sugar cravings, weight gain, diarrhea, constipation, hormonal imbalances, and even autoimmune disease. **But there are ways to check if you have leaky gut.**

The easiest way to check if you have leaky gut is to pay attention to your body and focus on how you feel, keeping an eye out for leaky gut syndrome symptoms. When in doubt, a leaky gut test will help address it quickly.

As a condition that has a thousand and one symptoms, determining whether or not you have leaky gut can be tricky. However, there are a few telling signs of a leaky gut which include:

- Developing new food sensitivities
- Asthma
- Inflammatory skin conditions such as acne, psoriasis, or eczema
- Irritable Bowel Syndrome (IBS) and Irritable Bowel Disease (IBD)
- Autoimmune disease
- Hormone imbalances such as low thyroid
- Mood disorders such as depression

Still not 100% sure if your symptoms are caused by leaky gut? You may want to take a leaky gut test. At present, one of the most effective ways to test for leaky gut is by doing a zonulin test.

Zonulin is a type of protein that regulates the size of the openings in your intestinal wall. Under normal circumstances, we require small openings in our gut lining for nutrient transport. However, high levels of zonulin can enlarge these openings, which leads to a leaky gut. A zonulin test will be able to detect whether or not you have elevated zonulin levels.

Zonulin test can be done by using an enzyme-linked immunosorbent assay test (ELISA) performed by a professional healthcare worker.

In addition, taking a food sensitivity or allergy test can also be helpful for determining whether or not you have leaky gut, as food sensitivities and allergies can develop from increased intestinal permeability.

Say you've got yourself a test and you've addressed that you have leaky gut. Good! You know what the problems are. You also know it's not uncommon. And while it might be tempting to ignore it for now and fix it later, you should not take leaky gut lightly. Here's why.

As mentioned above, symptoms of leaky gut can range from digestive discomfort and food sensitivities to full blown autoimmune disease. In fact, leaky gut has been linked to celiac disease, rheumatoid arthritis, Crohn's disease, colitis, irritable bowel syndrome (IBS), fibromyalgia, multiple sclerosis (MS), autism, cancer... and the list goes on.

There are a couple of reasons that leaky gut is associated with chronic illness.

Reason #1: Approximately 70% of your immune system cells are found in your gut.

Reason #2: The chronic inflammation caused by leaky gut is what can lead to inflammatory disease.

As you can see, leaky gut isn't a condition to ignore or take lightly. The good news is that leaky gut can be healed, and we will tell you how.

But in order to heal leaky gut, you need to be aware of what causes it first so that you can not only heal it but also prevent your gut from leaking ever again. **And what exactly causes leaky gut?**

Today's Western diet is full of pro-inflammatory foods that when frequently consumed can damage the cells in your gut tissue, called epithelial tissue, and promote intestinal permeability. These foods include:

- Corn
- Conventional dairy
- Soy
- Wheat and gluten
- Highly processed vegetable oils
- Refined Sugar
- Additives and preservatives found in processed foods

What To Do: Be aware that these foods are not good for your gut and replace them with healthier alternatives such as gluten-free grains, coconut oil, and nut or seed milk. By doing that, you'll begin to naturally reduce the inflammation in your Gastrointestinal tract (GI tract), which may help alleviate symptoms of leaky gut.

Food isn't the only source of inflammation in our lifestyles. A constant high level of stress can weaken your immune system, and a weakened immune system cannot do a good job of fighting off foreign invaders like bad bacteria and viruses, which can lead to inflammation and leaky gut.

What to Do: This one is obvious–reduce stress. In order to do that, we recommend the following:

- Get more sleep
- Add in some daily outdoor walks, which give you the opportunity to absorb vitamin D straight from the sun
- Do some activities that help you relax, such as yoga, swimming, and meditation
- Schedule some fun into your week
- Hang out with positive, inspiring, and uplifting people

A lack of beneficial gut bacteria is not a good thing. An imbalance of good bacteria and bad bacteria in your gut can cause leaky gut. The most common reasons for this imbalance are overuse of prescription antibiotic drugs and a lack of probiotics. Probiotics, in particular, are essential to preventing leaky gut, as they've been shown to help strengthen the gut barrier.

What To Do: Rebalance gut bacteria with probiotics by adding probiotic-rich foods to your diet. We bet that you already have some of the foods in your pantry. Go take a look and start adding them to your diet.

- Coconut yogurt
- Apple cider vinegar
- Raw cheese
- Fermented vegetables like kimchi, Sauerkraut, and salted gherkin pickles
- Brine-cured olives
- Japanese foods like miso, kombucha, and natto
- Kefir
- Tempeh

Toxic Overload: Believe it or not, we get exposed to heavy metals, household chemicals, environmental pollutants, additives, and preservatives every year. Those toxins are more common in our environment than ever before. When those toxins enter your body, your liver works extra hard to safely eliminate them. However, if you're constantly being exposed to these toxins, your liver can become overburdened, and your body's natural ability to detoxify slows down.

A sluggish digestive system can allow toxins to linger in your gut, which can contribute to damaging your gut lining, and therefore causing leaky gut.

What to Do: While you can't really control the amount of toxins you're exposed to, you can try to eliminate toxins as much as possible. That brings us to the simple steps to heal leaky gut.

Steps To Heal Leaky Gut: Now that you've learned about leaky gut from its syndrome to its cause and you've got a better idea of what to do and what not to do, we'd like to sum up the solution with 4 steps to keep you on track. In addition, we even created an actionable 5-day leaky gut diet plan using gut healing foods to make your gut healing process easy to start.

Avoid refined sugar, grains, processed foods, dairy, gluten and GMO foods. Other toxic exposures to eliminate include pesticides, NSAIDS, and antibiotics. It is recommended that you consult with your physician if he or she has prescribed these for you.

Even if you've been extra conscious about what you put in your mouth, you will not heal your gut if you are experiencing chronic stress. Often times, when we talk about stress, it's emotional. It could come from a crappy job or an unpleasant relationship.

We've recommended a few things to help reduce chronic stress like getting more sleep, taking walks under the sun, practicing yoga, and meditating. What's going to help more is to take a step back and reflect how everything is working out in your life. Pay attention and identify what constantly makes you stress out and decide if you need a change.

While good food is medicine, taking specific supplements in addition to a leaky gut diet may help accelerate the gut healing and take your health to the next level.

There are **many supplements** you can take. For any program that's designed to heal a leaky gut, L-glutamine is crucial.

L-glutamine is an amino acid that occurs naturally in your body and is synthesized in your muscles. While it contributes to your overall health in countless ways, L-glutamine has been shown to play an especially crucial role in intestinal repair.

- **It keeps your gut lining strong.** L-glutamine nourishes your epithelial cells, which are located in both your small and large intestine. This helps strengthen your gut lining and prevent it from breaking down and becoming permeable.
- **It rebuilds and repairs your gut lining.** In cases where the leaky gut is already present, L-glutamine has been shown to help counteract intestinal damage by rebuilding and repairing the

gut lining and protecting intestinal mucosa. The intestinal mucosa has been described as the body's "second skin", and plays a critical role in preventing pathogens from entering your gut barrier.

You can find L-glutamine supplements in both capsule and powdered form. Glutamine powder is an essential amino acid supplement that is anti-inflammatory and necessary for the growth and repair of your intestinal lining. It's recommended to take 2-5 grams twice per day.

Additionally, probiotics, digestive enzymes, and plant-derived mineral supplements can also contribute to effective gut healing.

Since certain foods are a rich source of L-glutamine and certain foods contains a high level of probiotics, we believe that the best way to consume these important items is to incorporate them into your diet. Now, the question is what foods can help heal leaky gut?

We've covered a few probiotic-rich foods before. On top of that, there are some foods that are rich in L-glutamine, amino acids, minerals which are essential to gut healing. We've done an in-depth study on leaky gut foods and identified what to eat and avoid in order to heal leaky gut and explained why in great detail in this study. In a nutshell, the best foods to eat are:

- **Bone Broth–** made with 100% grass-fed organic beef bones, organic vegetables, and herbs
- **Steamed Vegetables–** non-starchy vegetables for easy digest
- **Fermented Vegetables–** sauerkraut, kimchi, gherkin pickles
- **Raw cultured dairy–** yogurt, coconut milk kefir
- **Grass-fed meats–** beef, chicken, turkey and bison
- **Healthy fats–**avocado, coconut oil, salmon, tuna, egg yolk

For animal products, we recommend that you choose organic, grass-fed, wild and pasture raised animal products whenever possible. Organic, free range animal products will contain fewer hormones and antibiotics than farmed animals. Farmed animals have been shown to contain higher levels of hormones and antibiotics, which act as toxins that may contribute to damaging the gut lining.

By gradually reducing the amount of inflammatory foods in your diet, managing stress, and eating gut supportive nutrients each and every day, your gut health will quickly improve so you can live a life feeling your absolute best.

Please remember. to approach the health changes gradually. Keep it simple. If I had to start all over again, I would immediately start with the baking soda protocol, along with the essiac tea and intensive juicing. To obtain the cannabis oil might take a bit of time but please don't be afraid to throw everything at the cancer disease. Chaga tea is also renowned for its anti cancer properties. Also try a wonderful drink of garlic juice and ginger juice mixed with unpasturized honey and lemon juice. This is a drink that kills bronchitis. I know this from experienced. What the doctor prescribed did not work.

Recipe: One clove of garlic squeezed or grated.

One measure of ginger squeezed or grated.

Juice of half a lemon.

One half teaspoonful of raw-un-pasteurized honey.

Above is just a general outline but be free to experiment. Do what is best for you.

Boil one cup of water. Add the lemon juice, garlic, ginger and the honey. If you have bronchitis, you will experience a great improvement in the first few days. Drink three cups daily and keep the protocol going and you will see the bronchitis disappear. It worked for me when all the prescribed drugs and puffers did not work. It also cleans the kidneys, liver and colon. It is a wonder drink. You can add cayenne pepper for an extra kick, if you wish. Nature, really, has the answer to our woes.

Other books By John Gabriel

A Life Almost Wasted

A Waste of a Human Being

Paranormal

Desiderata

Go placidly amidst the noise and haste, and remember what peace there may be in silence. As far as possible without

surrender be on good terms with all persons;

Speak your truth quietly and clearly; and listen to others, even the dull and the ignorant; they too have their story.

Avoid loud and aggressive persons; they are vexations to the spirit. If you compare yourself with others, you may become vain or bitter; for always there will be greater and lesser persons than yourself.

Enjoy your achievements as well as your plans. Keep interested in your own career, however humble; it is a real possession in the changing fortunes of time.

ᴧse caution in your business affairs; for ᴧne world is full of trickery, but let this not blind you to what virtue there is; many persons strive for high ideals; and everywhere life is full of heroism.

Be yourself. Especially, do not feign affection. Neither be cynical about love; for in the face of all aridity and disenchantment it is as perennial as the grass.
Take kindly the counsel of the years, gracefully surrendering the things of youth.

Nurture strength of spirit to shield you in sudden misfortune. But do not distress yourself with dark imaginings. Many fears are born of fatigue and loneliness.

Beyond a wholesome discipline, be gentle with yourself. You are a child of the universe, no less than the trees and the stars; you have a right to be here.

And whether or not it is clear to you, no doubt the universe is unfolding as it should. Therefore be at peace with God, whatever you conceive Him to be, and whatever your labors and aspirations, in the noisy confusion of life keep peace with your soul.

With all its sham, drudgery, and broken dreams, it is still a beautiful world. Be cheerful.

Strive to be happy. ~ Max Ehrmann

John Gabriel

27055374R00094

Printed in Great Britain
by Amazon